ANDY WEST

The Life Inside

A Memoir of Prison, Family and Learning to be Free

PICADOR

First published in paperback 2022 by Picador

This edition first published 2023 by Picador
an imprint of Pan Macmillan
The Smithson, 6 Briset Street, London EC1M 5NR
EU representative: Macmillan Publishers Ireland Ltd, 1st Floor,
The Liffey Trust Centre, 117–126 Sheriff Street Upper,
Dublin 1 D01 YC43
Associated companies throughout the world

ISBN 978-1-0374-1201-1

Copyright © Andy West 2022

The right of Andy West to be identified as the
author of this work has been asserted in accordance
with the Copyright, Designs and Patents Act 1988.

All rights reserved. No part of this publication may be reproduced,
stored in a retrieval system, or transmitted, in any form, or by any means
(including, without limitation, electronic, mechanical, photocopying,
recording or otherwise) without the prior written permission of the publisher.

Pan Macmillan does not have any control over, or any responsibility for,
any author or third-party websites websites (including, without limitation,
URLs, emails and QR codes) referred to in or on this book.

1 3 5 7 9 8 6 4 2

A CIP catalogue record for this book is available from the British Library.

Typeset in Dante MT Std by Palimpsest Book Production Ltd, Falkirk, Stirlingshire
Printed and bound in the UK using 100% Renewable Electricity by CPI Group (UK) Ltd

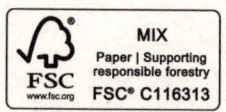

This book is sold subject to the condition that it shall not, by way of
trade or otherwise, be lent, hired out, or otherwise circulated without
the publisher's prior consent in any form of binding or cover other than
that in which it is published and without a similar condition including
this condition being imposed on the subsequent purchaser. The publisher does
not authorize the use or reproduction of any part of this book in any manner
for the purpose of training artificial intelligence technologies or systems.
The publisher expressly reserves this book from the Text and Data Mining
exception in accordance with Article 4(3) of the European Union
Digital Single Market Directive 2019/790.

Visit **www.picador.com** to read more about all our books
and to buy them.

An *Irish Times* and the *i* Book of 2022

'Insightful and sophisticated'
The TLS

'Tense and intimate . . . an education'
Geoff Dyer

'Written with sensitivity and humanity . . . a remarkable insight into prison life'
Amanda Brown, author of *The Prison Doctor*

'Authentic, fascinating and deeply moving'
Terry Waite

'Enriching, sobering and at times heartrending . . . a wonder'
Sir Lenny Henry

'Inspiring' *The Observer*

'Strives with humour and compassion to understand the phenomenon of prison'
Sydney Review of Books

'A fascinating and enlightening journey . . . A legitimate page-turner' 3:AM

'An honest, delicate memoir . . . I'll never think about prisons the same way again'
Ciaran Thapar, author of *Cut Short*

'West powerfully interweaves an account of teaching philosophy in prison with his own family's history of imprisonment, creating an intellectually thrilling memoir of freedom and constraint'
Alex Marzano-Lesnevich, author of *The Fact of a Body*

'Beautifully written – honest, painful, absurd and sometimes joyful'
Caitlin Davies, author of *Queens of the Underworld*

'A book that every thinking person should read'
Simon Critchley, author of *Continental Philosophy*

'An astonishingly necessary book . . . brilliantly dispels damaging myths about those whose lives are lived inside'
Lucia Osborne-Crowley

'More and more compelling with every turn of the page'
Erwin James, author of *Redeemable*

'Written with compassion and searing honesty'
The Tablet

'An incredible feat of thoughtfulness . . . a work that's both humane and unflinching'
Eleanor Gordon-Smith, author of *Illogical Stories*

'These are tender, complicated relationships, and there is candour and wisdom – and no little courage – in how West shows them to us'
New Humanist

'Immersing, entertaining and wonderfully empathetic'
The Bookseller

'The strength of West's storytelling lies in [this] personal narrative ... a blueprint for how to cope with the harsh and imposing logic of the justice system' PEN America

'Sets out the reality of doing time in Britain' *The Economist*

'One of the best books I've read this year. Moving, witty and profound, it's a powerfully humane book about a part of life that's defined by inhumanity' Matt Rowland Hill

'Drawn with great tenderness' *Prospect*

'This thoughtful debut ... tells a deeply personal story – full of struggle, insight and dark humour – through the lens of philosophy and West's compelling conversations with prisoners' *Morning Star*

'Anyone who is interested in thinking philosophically about complex family relationships will find much to ponder ... poignant, insightful, and full of philosophical substance'
The Philosophers' Magazine

'Brilliantly captures the boredom and frustration of jail ... both fascinating and moving' PressReader

'*The Life Inside* is extraordinary: at once a work of great moral searching that eloquently contemplates guilt, shame, redemption and the UK prison system, and an autobiographical investigation conducted with the utmost urgency'
Rob Doyle

Andy West has taught philosophy in over twenty prisons since 2016. His writing has featured in *The Guardian, The Telegraph, The Evening Standard, The Big Issue, Aeon,* 3AM Magazine and Huck. He was executive producer of the acclaimed BBC One series *Waiting for the Out* and Writer in Residence at HMP Grendon.

For my brother

Ideas are substitutes for griefs
  MARCEL PROUST

By my guilt I further gained the
right to intelligence
  JEAN GENET

Author's Note

Names and details of people, places and events have been changed or merged. Events have also been moved around in time. I have done this to protect privacy, maintain sensitivity towards victims, avoid compromising both prison and personal security and narrativize my experiences into a personal story. There is no such thing as the prison or the prisoner. There are a multitude of prisons and each person in prison has their own experience. Whilst this book aims to capture something of that plurality, it is foremost written from my subjective viewpoint as someone who had family in prison and now teaches inside. Classroom dialogues are drawn from a period of four years; I've tried to render the essence of the conversations, even when I wasn't able to recall what was said word for word. I have written my personal experiences as I remember them, and where possible I have done research or conferred with others to check the truthfulness of my memories. However, some may recollect things differently.

My students in prison are not allowed access to social media; they cannot publish anything in public without the Ministry of Justice's permission and many of them have difficulties writing. A lot of them live with a social stigma, which often means their voices are not heard or that they may not wish to talk about their experience if that means outing themselves as a prisoner or ex-prisoner. As I worked on this book, I was aware that I was writing about people who often don't have the chance to write about themselves. Everyone has stories to tell but only some are afforded the privilege to share stories with a larger audience. I have tried to remain mindful of the responsibility that comes with the opportunity that has been given to me. Where necessary, I have consulted ex-prisoners, colleagues and academics to check my understanding.

Thank you to my relatives who have entrusted me with telling their stories. I hope I have succeeded in writing about them with honesty and care.

Contents

Identity 1
Freedom 4
Shame 13
Desire 24
Luck 29
Happiness 53
Time 79
Madness 95
Trust 114
Salvation 135
Forgetting 159
Truth 166
Looking 182
Laughter 185
Race 203
Inside 222
Change 244
Stories 265
Home 287
Kindness 308

Classroom Materials and Sources 335
Acknowledgements 337

Identity

> Justice: to be ever ready to admit that another
> person is something quite different from what we
> read when he is there.
>
> Simone Weil

The man standing next to me inside the lift looks uncannily like my father, who I have not seen for twenty years, since he was sent to prison. He is short, has yellowed fingertips and the sleeves of his oversized suit jacket brush his knuckles. I have seen men who look like my father before, while I was on buses and trains or standing at urinals in pub toilets. I've seen them in London, Manchester, Berlin and Rio de Janeiro.

In the lift, I glance at him and I recognize the permanently clenched jaw, the emphysemic wheeze in the breathing. I pull my shirtsleeve over my wrist to conceal my watch and ask him for the time. He doesn't answer with a Scouse accent and therefore he's not my dad. Neither were the men in Germany or Brazil. We travel up another five floors in silence. The lift stops, the doors open and he exits.

Tomorrow morning I'll be going into a prison for the first time. I'll be teaching philosophy to men. A few months ago, I wrote a piece in the *Guardian* about teaching philosophy, where I mentioned that my dad, brother and uncle did time inside. Last month, a philosopher called Jamie from a local university asked me to co-teach in jail. I assume I have been invited to work on the project because I'll be a good fit culturally, because I might understand convict logic in a way that most *Tractatus*-clutching types wouldn't. Since Jamie asked me to work with them, I've been noticing a pair of heavy ankle-length black boots in a shop window. It's spring and I am in the habit of wearing soft leather Oxford shoes with stonewashed jeans twice rolled up at the bottom. This afternoon I went into the shop. They only had the boots in a size ten. I'm a size nine, but that doesn't matter to me so I bought them.

The next morning in prison, Jamie and I have set the chairs up in a circle and wait for our students. The classroom doubles as an art room. It's like the art classrooms from my schooldays except there are bars on the windows, and the pencils and paintbrushes and anything else with a pointed end are kept in padlocked cupboards.

I look over the pages of our lesson plan on Locke's theory of identity. I imagine my dad trying to make sense of it, and with a pen I strike red lines through entire paragraphs. 'Keep it accessible,' I say to Jamie. 'There's going to be a lot of illiterate guys, men who didn't finish school. Don't overwhelm them.' I hear the clanking of heavy metal doors being opened and the echoing voices of men talking in the corridor outside. Our students are approaching. I'm wearing my new boots; the unworn toecaps have a first-day-at-school shininess.

A man comes to the door. 'Is this psychology?' He has morning breath and bloodshot eyes.

'Philosophy,' I say.

He shrugs, walks in and takes a seat.

Another man comes in, gives me a bone-crushing handshake and looks past my shoulder. Another with sallow skin and receding gums. A man clutching a plastic bag with 'Leeds

University' printed on it; the bag is split at the seam but he still carries his library books in it. A man with a round face who looks skeletal in the photo of his ID card. I walk around the group introducing myself but wince at a pain in my feet. My boots are rubbing my skin. I feel the sting of fresh blisters on my heels. More men arrive until there are twelve. Jamie and I take a last look through our notes for today's class. 'Accessible,' I say again.

The men sit in a circle and I explain Locke.

'That's not quite right,' says a student called Macca.

'Excuse me,' I say.

'Locke didn't only care about memory.' He points at my whiteboard. 'It was more consciousness.'

All twelve men are looking at me. I walk over to the whiteboard, tiptoeing to avoid the shooting pain on my heels, wipe out the word 'memory' and write 'consciousness'. The men laugh and whisper to each other. I try to explain Locke again, moving only in small strides, careful not to land my whole foot on the floor. A few minutes later, another student, who has just finished a distance learning degree, explains how Rousseau might disagree with Locke. Twenty minutes in we have run out of material. From across the room, Jamie's eyes meet mine and the word 'accessible' silently rings out between us.

Jamie sets the students some work in small groups and suggests we go over to the desk in the corner of the room to confer. Jamie goes to the desk and I tiptoe behind.

Freedom

> Part of you may live alone inside,
>   like a stone at the bottom of a well.
> But the other part
>   must be so caught up
>   in the flurry of the world
>   that you shiver there inside
>   when outside, at forty days' distance, a leaf moves.
> Nâzim Hikmet

A few months on, I now wear the same soft leather Oxford shoes to prison every week that I wear most other days. I've just returned from three weeks travelling solo in Thailand. My skin has bronzed and my hair is caramel brown. I walk through the strip-lit corridors of the prison to my classroom. A man escorted by guards passes me from the opposite direction. He has a pallid forehead and flaking skin underneath his eyes. I roll down the sleeves of my shirt to hide my suntan. I get to the classroom and write the theme for today's lesson on the board: 'Freedom'.

Twenty minutes later, the officer outside in the corridor shouts, 'Free flow.' Free flow is the time the gates inside the prison are unlocked and men move from their cells to education, workshops or other activities. A few minutes later, the men arrive in my room. A forty-year-old called Zach walks in. He wears grey plimsolls that have Velcro straps. They are the shoes the prison issue to men when they don't have their own. His jumper is pushed up to his elbows, showing dozens of horizontal scars down the top of his forearm. Zach was due to have a parole hearing last month, but the day before it took place he punched a healthcare worker in the face.

A few other men trickle in. A student called Junior appears in the doorway. He's tall and wears a baby pink muscle shirt, showing off his round shoulders and pecs. He wears a fresh pair of Nike exclusive trainers. A few weeks ago, another man asked Junior what he was in for. He answered, 'I'm an entrepreneur.'

He steps into the class and shakes my hand. 'A pleasure to be back, sir,' he says. His voice is sonorous. His plucked eyebrows are rounded at the ends. He walks into the room, shakes everyone's hand whilst looking them in the eye and calls them 'sir'.

Junior takes the seat next to Zach and stretches his legs wide apart. Zach crosses his arms across his belly.

Wallace is the last person to arrive. He walks upright, not with his chest puffed out but confident in the protection his barrel-shaped body gives him. He takes the seat next to Junior but doesn't say anything to him. Wallace doesn't engage with most people. He's sixteen years into a twenty-year sentence. He doesn't use the gym but prefers to work out alone in his cell. Every day he writes a letter to his son.

Free flow finishes. I close the door.

I sit in the circle with the men. I say, 'In Homer's epic, Odysseus was captaining his ship back from the war in Troy to his home, Ithaca. But he was about to encounter the Sirens. The Sirens were half-human, half-bird creatures who lived on the rocks in the middle of the sea. They sang a song so beautiful that any man who heard it became drunk with love and jumped overboard to swim to the source of the sound. The Sirens fed on delirious sailors.'

'No man has ever heard the Sirens and lived to tell the tale,' I say. 'Odysseus orders his crew to put wax in their ears, so they don't fall under the spell. Sailors will be able to go about their ordinary business, preparing food, organizing the ropes.'

I say, 'But someone would need to be able to hear when the music had stopped, in case the men take the wax out of their ears too early. Odysseus gets his men to tie him to the mast. He'll be able to hear the song without jumping overboard. He tells his crew to ignore any demand he makes to be untied.

'They set sail. Odysseus hears the music. It reaches into him and holds him. He's flooded with desire and begs to be untied, but the crew just carry on with their daily duties. One man has been at sea so long that his homesickness has turned to numbness. He sees how passionate Odysseus looks. The sailor stops what he is doing and wants to know what the Sirens sound like. He takes the wax out of his ears. He becomes intoxicated and jumps overboard to his death.

'They pass the Sirens and Odysseus is untied. From that day on, he carries a pain in his heart because he will never again hear anything as beautiful as the Sirens' song.'

'The Sirens are crack,' Zach says. 'They even live on the rocks.'

The men laugh, except for Wallace.

I ask: 'There were the men with wax in their ears, Odysseus, and the man who took the wax out. Which man was the most free?'

I pass Wallace the hand-sized bean bag I use as a talking stick.

'The men with wax in their ears, they're the most free,' he says. 'They just get on with it. It's like us in here, we don't have to do things like pay bills or do the school run. I got freedoms they ain't got.'

'Like what?' I ask.

'I'm free from choice. Just like the man with the wax in his ears,' Wallace says.

Junior leans forward in his chair and says to Wallace, 'But if you don't have choice, you're not free.'

'Outside there's too many ways to get in trouble. In here, I can focus,' Wallace says.

A moment later, I ask Junior, 'Which man do you think is free?'

'Odysseus,' Junior says. 'He's the king. People have to do what he says.'

'But Odysseus is the most trapped a person can be,' Wallace says. 'No matter how good his experience is, he's always hankering for it to be better and no experience will ever be enough.'

'But Odysseus has done something with his life,' Junior says.

'Every time he remembers what he's done, he's going to feel tormented. You're more free in a cell,' Wallace says.

'The reason the men with wax in their ears aren't hurting like Odysseus is because they've never done anything with their lives. They're foot soldiers,' Junior says.

'They're keeping their heads down so that they can do what they need to do to get home,' Wallace says.

'What's the point in them getting home if that's how they're gonna live?' Junior says.

I hand a student called Keith the bean bag. He rests it on his lap and says, 'Now – there are several ways of looking at this.'

When I first started in prison, the librarian told me that Keith is thirteen years into his sentence, lives in a single cell and goes through a book every two or three days. Keith has a thick working-class Glaswegian accent and casually uses words like 'nomenclature'. 'You could look at it from a neuroscientific perspective,' he says. He talks with the speed that autodidacts often do, as if to unburden himself from his own mind, but other students are beginning to slump and stare at the floor.

'The one who jumps off is free like how in Shakespeare the jester is free in a way that the king isn't,' he continues. I want to interrupt him. I would love to interrupt him. For me, interrupting people is one of the perks of being a teacher. Outside of my professional life, I'm a soft-voiced and slow-speaking person who is forever being interrupted by loud, fast-talking people, and one reason I teach is so I can legitimately interrupt people and exact revenge for this. Keith continues: 'Quantum physics tells us that things aren't actually determined,' but I am unable to interrupt him. How do you say 'I'm aware of the time' to a man who has lived in a cell for thirteen years?

Eventually, Keith gives me back the bag. Zach has the sleeves of his jumper pulled down over his hands. I ask him what he thinks.

'The man who jumped off the ship,' Zach says.

'He was under a spell. He can't be free,' Junior says.

'But maybe it took courage to give in to the pull of the Sirens. Maybe he was the only one brave enough to take his freedom,' Zach says.

'He wanted to escape, but what he did is like escaping your cell and climbing onto the roof. Where do you go from there? You're more fucked than you were in your cell.'

'He jumped off because he realized that was the most free he could be in his situation,' Zach says.

'He jumped off because he gave up on freedom,' Junior says.

An hour into the class, it is time for the men to take a break to stretch their legs. I open my classroom door, but an officer in the corridor outside tells me I must shut it and keep everybody inside. There has been an incident on one of the landings where the cells are. A man has jumped onto the nets as a protest. Metal nets separate one floor of the prison landing from the one below. They stop people from dropping objects from above or from jumping to take their own life. When a man jumps onto one of these nets, security officers cannot go on and get them, for safety reasons. If they can't talk the man into coming off the nets, they must send in a special tornado team, clad in helmets and shields.

The officer tells me the man on the nets is imminently due to be deported to Venezuela to serve his sentence in prison there. He doesn't want to go. He has jumped on the nets to buy himself more time in this prison.

I shut my door and lock it. We take our fifteen-minute break in the classroom. Zach reaches through the bars on the window and opens it a few inches. Junior has gone to the whiteboard and used one of my pens to draw a diagram explaining to four men how to become a bitcoin millionaire. He's telling them what they need to do to afford a Rolex or Mercedes in the next six months.

A man called Gregg comes up to me. He has a bright scar striking through his ginger stubble. 'This philosophy. What's it for?' he asks.

'Well,' I say, 'philosophy is ancient Greek for—'

'What can you do with it? What jobs?'

'Some friends, some people I know, they work in the City now, I think.'

'What job do you have?' he says.

That he asks this immediately after I've taught him makes me think the answer 'philosophy teacher' isn't going to count. 'Some people do law conversion courses after a philosophy degree.'

Gregg stares at me expectantly, as if I am a man who has only said half of what he has to say.

'Who do you think is the most free in the Sirens story?' I ask.

'None of them. That's why it's called free-dumb. Only an idiot would believe in free-dumb.'

Wallace stays in his chair and doesn't speak to anybody for the whole fifteen minutes of the break. A few weeks ago, there was a security issue in prison and the men had to spend twenty-three hours a day in their cells, leaving only one hour for what the regime calls 'association' – the time where men are allowed out of their cells to make calls, shower, socialize and stretch their legs. Very often when association was called, Wallace stayed in his cell, lying on his bed, reading a book.

The men take their seats in the circle again.

I say, 'The philosopher Epictetus was born into slavery, but he believed that on a fundamental level, he was still free. He said that chains constrained his body but not his ability to choose.'

'You can still be free in your mind,' Wallace says.

I say, 'Epictetus believed you could learn to be free by first understanding what you can and can't control.'

'Each night when the screws are coming around to lock our cells for the night, I close my door before the screw has the chance to,' Wallace says.

'For control?' I ask.

'The same reason I always finish a phone call a minute before the screws say we have to hang up,' Wallace says.

'What happens if you don't?' I ask.

'I'll do something I'll regret. A few years ago, I saw a man talking on the phone after the screw had told him to hang up. An officer put his finger on the receiver. If that happened to me, I know that I'd punch someone. So I never let myself get in that situation. I hang up early.'

'Is that freedom?' I say.

'It keeps things simple,' Wallace says.

Half an hour later, a guard outside the door shouts, 'Free flow,' signalling the end of the lesson. I open the door and most of the men shuffle out, but a few linger. One points at my suntanned face and asks me where I have been. I try to keep my answers as clipped as possible, worrying that a group of jailed men might smart from hearing about Phuket's tropical beaches and full moon parties. But they keep asking me for more information. 'Did you go snorkelling?' 'What was your favourite part?' 'Would you ever move there?' Then one says flatly, 'Did you go with your boyfriend?'

I search his face for a smirk. But there isn't one. He's being sincere. 'I was alone this time,' I say.

The men keep asking me questions about Thailand. A few have been themselves and want to know if this or that karaoke bar is still open in Bangkok. They ask if I got a good deal on flights, if I got the shits while I was there. As I answer their questions, I consider dropping into the conversation that I have a girlfriend, but the atmosphere in the room now is so genial and tolerant that I don't have the heart to tell them I'm not gay.

Shame

'But I'm not guilty,' said K., 'there's been a mistake. How is it even possible for someone to be guilty? We're all human beings here, one like the other.'

'That is true,' said the priest, 'but that is how the guilty speak.'

FRANZ KAFKA

Tonight, I do my online tax return. I click the Complete button and immediately feel depressed. I go to bed but cannot sleep. I'm certain that I have done it wrong, have underpaid, and that I will be prosecuted.

In my sleep, I dream I'm in a prison yard with my father. I am side-on to him. I step away, mindful that I don't want the guards to see us together. It is a winter afternoon and I am cold. Two prison guards are laughing and joking with each other. I go up to them and tell them that I work here and that I'll be leaving the prison with them at the end of the workday. They continue talking with each other as if they cannot hear me. I reach for my keys, but my key pouch is empty. I ask the guards if they can hear me, but they do not respond.

I wake up at five o'clock with the sunrise. Heavy rain falls sideways and I leave the house without my umbrella to walk to prison. The backs of my ears and neck are wet. I arrive at the prison's security gate, take off my soaked shoes, watch and belt and walk through the metal detector, feeling the hard floor through my wet socks. I feel faint and my heart races. I'm in the grip of wild, irrational guilt. My rucksack passes through an X-ray machine. The security officer gives me a stern look and working backwards from it to what my crime might be, I imagine the light on the scanner is about to go red and beep and the guards will find a kilo of heroin in my bag.

The alarm doesn't beep. I hold my arms out limply to be searched by the security officer, the sleeves of my jumper damp. I pass security, but that doesn't exonerate me from the panic. I go through the prison grounds, past a wall with rows of cell windows and hear the sound of multiple televisions all at once. Yoghurt advert jingles. Emergency news reports. Canned laughter.

It's been several years since I have had this paranoia that the sins of my father will be handed down to me no matter what choices I myself make. The grim assuredness that I'd go to prison was strongest when I was eighteen and I used to worry not if I would get arrested but how. I hoped it would happen in the daylight rather than at night, when I was alone rather than with friends. I'd become distracted when I heard police sirens, pausing to try and tell if they were getting closer. In the corridor of the prison, an officer holding an Alsatian on a leash comes from the other way, and I slow my pace as if to invite the dog to bark at me. It passes, staring at me with its black eyes.

My student David won't be able to attend today because he has a legal visit, so at lunchtime I go to his cell before class to give him some reading. His cellmate opens the door and I'm hit by a smell. They have four purple air-fresheners on their windowsill, and the lavender has mixed with the smell of socks, cooked instant noodles and two men in a small space. He tells me David is still on lunch-serving duty. I go to the food-serving area where there is a long queue of men waiting in line and wonder if it might be better to come back later. I ask a man who looks to be about seventy what time lunch normally finishes. 'We was supposed to eat half hour ago,' he says. He has the same Liverpudlian accent as my father. 'I've asked them what time we was gonna have lunch and they said in a few minutes, and that was twenty fuckin' minutes ago. There's no such thing as time in this place.'

I leave David for later. I get to my classroom and find a woman is packing toys into a box. Teddy bears, Lego bricks, a rainbow-coloured xylophone and a Fisher-Price telephone with wheels and a smiling face on the front. She says she teaches the men how to play so they know what to do with their children on visit days.

She leaves. I set up the chairs in a circle and wait for the guards to call free flow.

A few years before I was born, my dad went to prison for eighteen months. He continued to be in trouble with the law throughout my childhood. When I was two, Mum, Dad and I went on holiday to Jersey. I was too young to remember it myself, but Mum says that on the second night of the holiday, my dad became jealous of a handsome waiter who was being polite to Mum. Mum and I went back to the hotel. Dad stayed out drinking. At 1 a.m., he staggered through the door and threw a handful of jewellery at her feet. There were gold rings and diamond earrings.

'There you go,' Dad said, his alcoholic breath in her face.

'What have you done?' Mum said.

They heard the sound of police sirens approaching. Dad stood there with a pearl necklace caught dangling on his fingers.

He had smashed the window of a jewellery shop and taken handfuls of goods from the display. A few minutes later, the police arrived and arrested him. He appeared in court the next day. He'd have been going back to prison again were it not for the fact that the gold, diamonds and pearls he'd taken were plastic display versions of the real thing. The judge found him guilty of property damage and ordered him to pay a fine. Mum handed over the rest of the holiday money. She adjusted our tickets and we travelled home that day.

Dad didn't want neighbours to find out that we'd come back early, or else they might start asking why. For the rest of the week, we stayed inside with the curtains closed.

When I was seven, my parents broke up, and Dad moved to a place a thirty-minute drive away. He got a job as an insurance salesman. I stayed with him every other weekend, playing with the other kids who lived on the street. Eighteen months later, on a Sunday, around midday, the phone rang. Dad was still in bed. The phone went onto the answer machine and I heard an old man accusing Dad of defrauding him out of thousands of pounds.

Two weeks later, Dad picked me up from school and drove me for four hours to his new home. I passed the time by looking out of the window and counting the motorway lights until I got to a thousand and when I reached a thousand I started again from one and counted a thousand more. We arrived at a seaside town where he was renting a top-floor studio flat.

At night, we went to the pub. He quickly got drunk. He introduced himself to the barmaids and other punters under a fake name. We sat at a table in the corner. I bit my nails, twiddled my hair with my fingers and kept fidgeting.

'Sit still,' he said.

I put my hands on my lap. I felt sick with nervousness.

He nudged me and nodded towards two burly men at the bar. 'If anyone in here tries to touch me, those blokes will step in. They're my minders.' But the two men didn't pay him any notice at all. Dad necked another drink and said to me, 'If anyone talks to you, don't tell them where we used to live before.'

In his flat, he hadn't put any pictures on the walls. Instead of a table, there was an unfolded ironing board at the end of his bed that he kept his things on. Pens, cigarette lighters, a reel of Sellotape, keys, a comb, small cartons of UHT milk, a half-eaten bag of fizzy sweets, and the names of racehorses scribbled on the bottom of takeaway menus. He'd drink at night and sleep until late in the morning. I sat close to the TV, watching cartoons on the quietest volume. He jumped in his sleep and shouted out 'No!' before rolling over and going back to sleep.

I watched cartoons to try and distract myself from the block of tension in my chest. They finished at about midday. I flicked through the channels but all the programmes were for adults. I sat on the windowsill and looked at people passing by in the street below.

In the afternoon Dad wanted to play-fight with me. He knelt down so that his face was in front of mine.

'Hit me,' he said.

He turned his head to the side and pointed at his jaw.

'Hit me. Come on,' he said.

I held my hands by my side.

He slapped his jaw.

'Come on. Hit me,' he said.

I kept my arms by my side.

We went to the pub. He put a drop of his beer in my lemonade and told me I should try it. But I left my glass on the table. I wanted to make sure I wasn't like him but I already felt ashamed that I was. On Monday morning, when he dropped me back at school, I walked into my classroom with a feeling of dread that I was in trouble for something. When my teachers were friendly and welcoming to me, the guilt didn't lift. I had to keep it inside me, like a secret. When the religious studies teacher told us about the saints in heaven, I asked him what kind of people go to hell.

Nine months later, Dad moved again, an hour down the road from the last place. When we met people, he introduced himself to them under a new fake name. This time he was living in a caravan. At night we unfolded the sofa into a bed and topped-and-tailed. He slept with a baseball bat beside his pillow. I became more and more tense. I started obsessively worrying that I was somehow bad. Whilst Dad was sleeping, I knelt down and prayed to God to give me another chance to be a good person.

Six months later, Dad moved again; this time the place was a few hundred metres from a ferry port. He used a different fake name and still slept with his baseball bat beside his bed. His drinking got worse and he became more aggressive. At midday, he was still asleep. I knelt down and prayed. Outside, the ferries blew their horns as they were leaving.

When I was twelve, I was at Mum's house when I received a letter from my dad. He said he was in trouble with the police and his lawyer thought that he might be facing jail time again. I ended contact with him there. I changed my name so it was different from his. But the dread lingered.

One weekend when I was seventeen, my best friend Johnny and I were in town and I saw a red shirt in a shop that I wanted but couldn't afford. The next day, Johnny bought it for me as a gift. He handed it to me and I felt an obscure sense of guilt. In my mind, I imagined this was going to be the last time anyone was ever going to give me a gift because soon people would find out who I really was and they would no longer want to give me their friendship. I put the shirt on and I felt a desperate need to confess. I didn't have anything to confess, but that didn't make the need any less urgent.

It was as if I had an executioner in my head, ready to darken the moment. In my teens and early twenties, I couldn't stop anticipating how soon everything would be taken away from me. A day I spent on the beach with my friends was tinged with desperation, like the final meal before the chamber. I tried to remind myself that I had not in fact committed any crime for which I should feel guilty, but the executioner dealt me a Kafkaesque bind, whereby arguing for my innocence only confirmed I had something to hide. There was nothing I could say or do. It was too late.

Now I'm thirty-one and I still carry a sense of inherited guilt. Since I've been working in prisons, the executioner has become more oppressive. I see men in their cells and my body goes cold with the thought that their punishment could be – or should be – my own.

★

Free flow starts. Keith arrives, takes a seat and reads a book he has on symbolic logic. Someone lingers outside the door. It's Rodney, a man in his early twenties. A month ago, he was reading books on criminal law in his cell until he was told he had lost his right to appeal. He's now serving his sentence 400 miles away from his home in Glasgow.

He looks at me side-on. 'I'm not coming next week,' he says.

'I always like to have you here,' I say.

He shrugs. 'I'll come this week cos they unlocked us, but I won't come next week.'

Rodney has said this to me for the last three weeks.

'It's nice that you're here,' I say.

He steps into the room and takes a seat.

I close the door.

I tell the men, 'In the ancient Greek story, Zeus wanted to punish Prometheus and Epimetheus for giving the humans fire. He chained Prometheus to a mountain where birds came and pecked out his liver each day. Then, on Epimetheus's wedding day, Zeus gave Epimetheus's wife, Pandora, a beautiful jar, but he told her that she wasn't allowed to look inside. Over the following days, she couldn't stop thinking about what was in the jar, until one night she opened it. Seven evil spirits came out. Hatred, Shame, Greed, Boredom, Laziness, Delusion and Pain. A voice from inside the jar cried out to Pandora and she opened it again. This time Hope came out.'

Rodney rubs his eyes.

I ask the men, 'If you could put one back into the box, which one would you pick?'

'Hope,' Rodney says.

'Hope is what makes the other evils worse,' he says. 'Pain wouldn't be so bad if there wasn't hope. We'd just live with it instead of hoping we weren't in pain.'

'Without hope nothing changes,' Keith says. 'Without hope you'd still have pain. It would just be pain with despair.'

'If you hope for things to change and they don't, then hope has just made everything worse,' Rodney says.

My gaze falls on the spirals of barbed wire I see through the window. Coils of it on rooftops and walls, loops of it everywhere above you in the prison.

'Pain would be less painful without hope,' Rodney says, and my attention comes back to the room.

'Hope is the child of the other evils in the box. When you are in pain, hope is there to remind you there's a future beyond pain,' Keith says.

'I don't waste my energy hoping for pain to go away. I just try and get used to it,' Rodney says.

The discussion continues. I write a list of the things to come out of Pandora's Box on the whiteboard. Keith says, 'Last year I had a hearing and I'd done everything possible for them to let me out, every kind of course. My behaviour was perfect. I was a model prisoner. I'd hoped I'd get out. In the end, the hearing lasted about eight minutes. They said no. I went on hunger strike. I promised myself I wasn't going to hope for a release date again.'

Rodney yawns.

'But I couldn't do it,' Keith continues. 'Not hoping made me empty. I didn't have the energy to work out or talk to people. I felt too empty to sleep. After a few days, three kids on my landing noticed I hadn't been eating and they brought a plate up to my door. I couldn't help but start hoping again.'

'That's a nice story, but I'm not going to be the idiot who tries to swim upstream,' Rodney says.

'There are too many decent people around to not hope,' Keith says.

Rodney points at the list of evils on the board. 'If you put hope back in the box, you'd automatically lose delusion too.'

Over the next hour, more men share ideas. Rodney looks bored. Twice, he laughs to himself, but it's not clear what he finds funny. Another man, Ed, is doing a six-year sentence. He has a grey goatee and bald head. I ask him what he would put back in the box.

'Shame,' he murmurs.

'Then you'd just keep doing bad things,' Rodney says.

'I've known before I did bad things that I'd feel shame after doing them and I still did them anyway,' Ed says.

'You'd never learn to be good if you didn't feel shame about the bad stuff you do,' Rodney says.

'Maybe it's shame that makes you do bad things.'

'How the fuck you supposed to be good then?'

'Empathy, maybe. Remorse. Not shame.'

An hour later, the class ends and the men are filing out. I put my rucksack over my shoulder. Gregg has waited behind to tell me he won't be here next week because he's being let out. 'They gave me a job working on the underground railway,' he says.

'Driving a train?' I say.

He frowns. I sense I have just misunderstood something basic, again.

'Fixing the tracks at night. Criminal record don't matter there because there's no public around,' he says.

'How do you feel about it?'

'It's something.'

A knot twists in my stomach at the thought that one of the only 'somethings' for Gregg after prison is an underground place of physical labour.

Gregg says goodbye and leaves. I take off my rucksack and open it. I kneel down and feel around inside the pockets to check again I'm not carrying any illegal items.

Desire

> My dreams are a stupid shelter, like an umbrella against lightning.
>
> FERNANDO PESSOA

My students continue to think I'm gay. During a discussion on knowledge, a student called Marcus uses the term 'batty man', and the others shoot him an unamused look. Marcus looks over to me and says, 'Sorry, boss.' I give him a gentle and forgiving smile. I go on teaching in prison as a closet heterosexual. The students believing I'm gay seems to make them less threatened by me, and in turn I feel more at ease as their teacher.

The night before a class, Jamie and I photocopy some readings about Buddhist philosophy. Then we realize the pages we have photocopied have tantric images of gods and goddesses in ecstatic union against a blue sky. Security have told us that any images involving penetration are not allowed in the prison. An officer recently put posters on the walls of the landings that listed what kind of images would be classed as pornography and therefore deemed contraband. Men can have lingerie models on their cell walls provided no nipples are on show. No naked or revealed vaginas, women urinating, erect or semi-erect penises.

So we can make new photocopies purely of the text, Jamie and I get some scissors and frantically cut out the spiritual images; a confetti of phalluses and breasts flutter down across our desk.

Lying in bed, I google, 'Are conjugal visits allowed in UK prisons?' The answer is no.

A few weeks later, I arrive in the education block of the prison and find that my regular classroom is being used for a talk by a recruiter from a healthy fast-food chain that offers jobs to ex-prisoners. A towering security officer called Baxter, with a wide jaw, pockmarked cheeks and a forearm full of tattoos, tells me I'm to use Room Nine instead. I open the door to Room Nine and find tall bookshelves in the middle of it. The bookshelves are on wheels, so I grip the side of the shelves and try to push them, but they don't move. 'Are you OK?' I turn around and Baxter is in the doorway, offering to help. There's also a woman sitting at the desk in the classroom, who I've never spoken to but I know is called Anika.

'I got it,' I say to Baxter and he leaves.

Anika doesn't look up from the paperwork she is filling out.

'Sorry, I didn't realize you were here,' I say.

'OK,' she says, still not looking up. She has peroxide-blonde hair falling over one side of her face. I know her name because I'd seen her teaching in the prison before and asked a colleague what her name was. I think she is beautiful, as do all the other men in the building; men sent down for murder or arson behave like perfect gentlemen around Anika. I squat down, unclip the brakes on the bottom of the bookshelf wheels and then stand up and try to move the bookshelf again, but it's no less stuck than before.

'Excuse me,' I say.

Anika keeps her pen on the page and looks at me over the top of her glasses. 'I'm just wondering,' I say, 'if you know how these wheels work? I thought I'd unlocked them but the shelves still won't move.'

She takes off her glasses. 'If you unlock the wheels the shelves will move.'

'I must be doing it wrong.'

I see her leg is shaking in irritation under the desk. She has a pointed jaw and high cheekbones. Inside a men's prison, her already sharp beauty takes on a merciless quality. I look at her and I feel sorry for the hundreds of men yearning inside their cells. Which is to say, Anika looks at me – looks right through me – and I feel sorry for myself.

When my dad got into pub fights or trouble with the police, I saw how his girlfriends grew dissatisfied and weary, so I came to believe that what women most wanted wasn't tough guys but men who were soulful and sensitive. Using my shoulder, I press as hard as I can into the bookshelves, but they still don't budge.

Baxter is back at the door and this time says, 'Let's have a look!' as I step out of the way. He grips the bookshelves and moves them out of the way.

'Thank you, Officer,' Anika says. She sighs.

'Yeah. Thanks,' I say.

An hour later, the men are filing into my class. Rodney arrives and tells me that he will come this week but not next week, just like he has been saying for the last four weeks. There is a new student in the class called Jack, a former accountant in his late fifties who is in prison for the first time for what will be a six-year sentence. He wears owlish glasses and a bright turquoise polo shirt. The colour hasn't faded yet. He sits next to Solomon, who knows prison well. Jack is complaining that he hasn't been given a replacement battery for his radio. Solomon says, 'If anyone asks to buy your radio, come to me first. I know some people.'

I shut the door.

I say, 'Descartes asked this question: is there any way we can prove that we are not in a dream right now?'

Solomon says, 'If this is a dream, I'm gonna have a right go at myself when I wake up.' The rest of the men laugh.

'I know I'm not in a dream because I never dream I'm in prison,' Jack says.

'You haven't been here long enough yet,' Rodney says.

Solomon points at his own face with both hands and says, 'My dreams are still at home.'

'Jammy bastard,' Rodney says.

Solomon lifts his hands in the air, pouts and does a smug dance.

'I dreamt I was at home once,' Rodney says. 'When I tried to pick things up, my hand would just sink through them.'

I ask, 'How do you know you're not still in that dream? How do you know this is reality?'

'What's the difference exactly?' Solomon says. 'Years ago, I woke up in hospital and the doctor told me I'd fallen from my balcony. I couldn't remember it because I was high. I didn't even experience it when it was happening. Sometimes I get these dreams where I can feel myself falling. I can feel the air on my arms.'

'What do you think the difference is?' I ask.

Jack taps the middle of his glasses. 'Reality makes sense. All of this makes too much sense to be a dream. It's physical. I can touch the chair. I can touch my watch.'

'Dreams can be physical, big man,' Solomon says.

'Not physical-physical. Not like real life.'

'The other night,' Solomon says, 'man in my cell woke up screaming his woman's name and he was wet in his shorts. Said he had a dream that he was with her.' Solomon holds his hands out in front of him as if gripping something the shape of a watermelon. 'He could smell her and taste her. Feel her.'

A grin breaks out across my face and I look around the room to meet the eyes of another man, but the rest of the men are earnestly listening to Solomon. 'Dreams can be physical. Man had to get up and change his shorts.'

Ray leans back in his chair and strokes his chin.

'So,' I say, 'what does the wet dream mean for Descartes' question?'

Luck

> A man in a desert can hold absence in his
> cupped hands knowing it is something that feeds
> him more than water. There is a plant he knows
> of near El Taj, whose heart, if one cuts it out, is
> replaced with a fluid containing herbal goodness.
> Every morning one can drink the liquid the
> amount of a missing heart.
>
> Michael Ondaatje

Seven years ago, my older brother Jason moved into his new accommodation. He painted the walls with five coats of emulsion, even though they only needed about two. Jason said he wanted to make sure the place was completely white.

Three days later, I visited Jason and his place still stank of emulsion. I went around the flat opening the windows to let some air in. In his bedroom, I knelt on his mattress, leaned across to reach the window and opened it. I pushed myself off the bed and saw I'd ruffled the duvet.

I'd not known Jason to sleep on a bed for years. He'd fall asleep in an armchair, his head curling down towards his knee. But for the last 374 days, Jason had been making his bed before doing anything else in the morning. In rehab, he'd learnt to do hospital corners.

I picked at the edges of the duvet and smoothed down the covers.

I went into the living room, where there was a new cot

with a solar system mobile hung above it that Jason hadn't finished putting together. Saturn, Earth and Venus were still on the carpet. I sat on the sofa while Jason knelt on the floor, watching over his seven-month-old son next to him. Scott played with a small plastic yellow cup, squeezing his hand around it and letting go again.

I was twenty-four and Jason was thirty-six. But he used to look more aged than he was. His skin had been grey, but now his cheeks had a reddish glow. He was wearing a new pair of blue shorts. For the twenty years before that, he'd worn bootcut jeans and a parka coat that he wore zipped up to his chin even when it was thirty degrees. He had had bony legs that were lumpy from past abscesses, but now he was going to the gym and his calf muscles were becoming defined.

That day was the fourth time I'd seen Jason in four months. That was as much as I'd seen him in the previous four years. He had a suntan, which made the scars that peppered his body more pronounced. They were on his cheek, in his hairline, stubble and on his hands. When he lifted his T-shirt up, I saw one the shape of a pebble beneath his ribcage. I always needed to know how he got each of his scars. On that day, I noticed he had one running from an inch above his knee, upwards, disappearing at the line of his shorts. I tilted my head to look at it.

'How did you get that?' I asked.

Jason opened his leg out, pulled up his shorts and pointed to a smaller scar on the inside of his thigh. 'That's where it came out,' he said.

'Where what came out?'

'Looking back, I suppose it was half my fault. I was with

the wrong people. I woke up in a kitchen. It was three in the morning on a council estate. There was this Irish bloke and his dad. I owed them money. I could hear them sharpening the knife in one of those knife sharpener things. I was sobering up rapidly, remembering one of them saying "Get him in the back of the van." The two of them came towards me. There's no way I could fight them. I was too weak from the drugs. One of them said, "Where do you want to be stabbed?"'

My toes curled. I pinched my skin at the crease of my elbow to try and direct the tension into one place.

'I told them "nowhere". But one of them swooped the knife sideways and I tried to dodge it but fell back and landed on my arse. I was stuck between the cooker and fridge. I was shitting myself. I knew those two had shot and killed someone before. They'd do it messy if I fought back. So I told them my leg.'

Scott's hair was gathered up on his head like a coconut. Jason patted it down. He said to me, 'I don't like you hearing this sort of thing, Bruv. Why don't I put the little man's shoes on him and we can go to the park?'

'They stabbed you,' I said.

Jason picked up one of Scott's yellow cups off the floor and put it back in his son's lap. 'They bent down either side of me, took an arm each round their necks and lifted me up. I steadied myself on the counter. The dad swung the knife into my leg. The first thing I thought was fuck, I only just got these jeans last week.'

Scott came up onto his hands and knees and pensively rocked back and forth.

'It felt like being punched really hard. Not as bad as I imagined it would be. But then they left the knife in and one of them took a few steps back; he ran up and kicked the knife. I fell over going fuck fuck fuck fuck fuck.'

Jason put his hand in front of his mouth. 'Sorry, baby. Daddy shouldn't swear.' Jason turned to me and asked, 'Do you think he can pick that up?'

I said, 'How did you survive? Don't worry, Scott won't understand.'

He stroked Scott's cheek. 'I was screaming F, F, F. One of them said, "He'll wake everyone up." The dad opened the kitchen door onto the street. The other one gave the knife a wobble so it comes out the other side. I screamed again and one of them was telling the other to keep the noise down. They picked me off the floor, took me out into the street and left me there. I got my phone out to try and text but kept losing consciousness. I dropped the phone. On the other side of the car park I saw a bloke and a woman. I limped towards them shouting for help and fell onto the gravel. The bloke put his arm around her and went in the other direction. "Drunk" I heard him say.'

Scott squirmed and his face turned down. My brother picked him up, smelt his nappy. 'He's shit himself,' Jason said and reached across the floor for a baby bag with little blue animals on it.

'I managed to summon the energy to get up and hobble forward, my feet squelching cos my trainers were full of blood. I got to the towers and pressed every single intercom buzzer. My eyelids were warm and heavy. A hello came out the intercom. "I've been stabbed," I said. "Can you call an ambulance?" The voice said a load of stuff in something foreign. I said "Help! Ambulance. 999. I'm bleeding." I heard a clicking sound where they hung up.'

Jason laid Scott on a plastic mat and opened the buttons of his son's onesie. He took nappies and wipes out of the baby bag and put a fresh nappy underneath Scott.

'I was leaning against the wall. I hobbled towards this light I could see that was probably the petrol station, but I turned over on my ankle in an alleyway. I was in a heap on the floor. I tried to drag myself forward using my arms, but my hip bone scraped against the gravel. I lay there and closed my eyes. You know how they say your life flashes before you just before you die? I remembered things I hadn't thought about in years. I could feel myself drifting away.'

I felt queasy. The emulsion smelt overpowering again. Scott let out a cry. 'I know, baby,' Jason said, bending to touch his nose to his son's. Scott pawed his father's face and went quiet.

'Then there was this smell. I opened my eyes. I was lying right next to a dog shit. I thought, whatever happens, I'm not dying in dog shit. I got enough energy to crawl out onto the pavement. Next thing I remember is a bloke putting a blanket over me saying the ambulance will be here soon.'

Jason opened the tabs on the side of Scott's nappy, took it off and put it in a sanitary bag. I leaned back into the sofa, exhausted from the story.

Jason took out a baby wipe and wiped away shit from the fold of skin between Scott's leg and groin.

A fight on the wing has meant the officers could only transport two men to my class today. I sit across the table from Samson and Patrick. Samson has bags under his eyes and high eyebrows, so he looks both exhausted and perpetually surprised. The blue lines of his veins show through the pale skin of his temples. He hasn't said anything since the class started ten minutes ago. Tomorrow will be Patrick's thirtieth birthday. He's come back to prison two weeks ago after only two weeks out. His teeth are long from where his gums have receded from the heroin.

I say to the two men, 'Imagine there's two fictional worlds. In one of them, good things happen to good people and bad things happen to bad people. It's the Just World. In that world, people are responsible for where they are and get no more or no less than they deserve.'

'I agree. The problem is that most people don't think like that. They're too full of self-pity. Like in here, so many people whinging about why they don't deserve to be in prison,' Patrick says.

'In the other imaginary world, the Luck World, they might not get caught. Everything there is decided by a dice. Your income, education, mental health. Whether you're a judge sentencing people or you end up going to prison. Your life expectancy. In the Luck World, good things might happen to bad people one day and bad things the next, or not; it's totally down to chance. People aren't responsible for where they are.'

'You're right,' Patrick says. 'That world is imaginary.'

'So you think our world is more like the Just World than the Luck World,' I say.

'I'm in prison because I made a choice. I chose to put heroin in my body.' Patrick points his finger at his own neck.

I cannot see any living veins in his neck.

Patrick continues, 'It's easier to say you've been unlucky than to face up to your own immaturity.'

'What if people aren't to blame for their immaturity?' I ask.

'I'm thirty fucking years old and I still haven't grown up.

My little boy is gonna be seven this year. I can't keep coming to jail or else before I know it he's gonna be an adult,' Patrick says.

I look to Samson, but he stares into the middle distance.

I say, 'In the Luck World, they'd play Snakes and Ladders because whether you win or lose has nothing to do with your level of skill. It's completely a game of chance. In the Just World, they'd play chess because it has no random factors. The one who plays the best wins.'

I lean my elbows on the table. 'But what about us?' I say. 'Our lives are set on the murky borderlands between the Just World and the Luck World. Life is a game of skill, but it's also random.'

I look at Samson. He blinks once but doesn't return the look.

I say, 'We can only be responsible for the things we have control over, but most of who we are is shaped by things outside of our control. We don't decide if we have a traumatic childhood or an addictive personality.'

'Actions have consequences,' Patrick says. 'I'm sick of excuses. People chat shit about how they were unlucky to have had a bad childhood. I wanna say to them, "Your bad childhood didn't score heroin for you. You did." If I relapse, it's not bad luck they'll find in my piss test.'

'I think who we are is an accident. Each of us could have been anyone else,' I say.

'You can be someone else if you change your behaviour. If man wants to get away from crime, then stop wearing your hoodie and go and buy a fucking pair of chinos. If you do that, the mandem won't be interested in you no more. Get on with your life.'

'Some people are lucky enough to not have to worry about the mandem,' I say.

'If they look at you, then cross the road and walk past them.'

'So, life is a game with no random factors?' I say. 'Really?'

'I put myself in prison. Next time, I can keep myself out,' Patrick says.

I turn to Samson. He looks like he's somewhere else. I ask him, 'Is our world closer to the Luck World or the Just World?'

Staring straight forward, he says, 'I'm in here for causing death through dangerous driving. I don't know who I am any more. I killed someone, but I'm not a killer.'

An hour later, I'm walking through the landing and someone behind me shouts my name. I turn and see it's Osman, one of the men who should have been in my group today. We bump fists and I can smell jasmine and sandalwood. He's wearing attar, a perfume that the prison lists on the 'Islamic Products' section of the canteen sheet. Osman tells me he won't be coming to my class any more because he has a job in the kitchen. He has been on the waiting list for a kitchen job for almost a year. He has four years left on his sentence and my philosophy course is only ten weeks long. He needs something that offers a more long-term distraction.

'What was you debating today?' he asks.

'Luck,' I say.

'I don't know what that is.'

'You've never been lucky?'

'You'd have to ask someone else. I don't ever think about luck. Luck will have you looking out the window.'

'Never been unlucky?'

'I've been washing pots. Then drying up. Then putting away.' Osman laughs.

'And after that?'

'After that I come back the next day and I wash, dry and put away.'

I lived with my brother for the first part of my childhood. When he shaved his head, I wanted to shave my head. When he played a computer game, I wanted to play it too. When, to amuse himself, he told my mum I'd given the finger to a passing police car and called them 'cunts', I denied it and burst into tears. After I'd calmed down, he apologized.

'I only said it because that's something you'd never do,' he said.

'It's not funny,' I said.

In the second half of my childhood, I only saw Jason a few times a year. He was in prison and when he wasn't, his life was very chaotic. The night Jason got stabbed I would have been about fourteen and living with my stepfather. The son of an orphan, my stepfather was a hard-working double-glazing salesman who bought his own house. Whilst Jason was ringing the buzzers on the intercom hoping that someone would help him, I would have been asleep in my bed.

I missed Jason all the time. When I was a teenager I went to house parties and my friends offered me alcohol and drugs. I always refused. Getting high would have felt like I was saying that what Jason was going through wasn't real or didn't matter. I would leave just as the night was gaining momentum. On the walk home, any melancholy I felt about missing out was buried under something much bigger. Having lots of fun whilst my brother was inside would have made me feel like I was being obnoxious. I was teetotal, in dedication to Jason. It was a way to love him in his absence.

Jason thinks he probably went to prison about twelve times before becoming a father to Scott. Sometimes he was away for a matter of weeks. Other times he'd be away for eighteen months. Almost all of his convictions were for a drug-related crime. Once, in court, he was high and fell asleep on the stand. Another time, in the early hours of the morning, Jason was drunk and saw a police car driving down the street. He stepped into the road, kicked the car as it passed him and shouted 'Taxi.' The police didn't stop. Jason stood in the middle of the road watching the car drive away.

Jason first went inside when he was sixteen. A decade or so later, when I was sixteen, I was waiting for him on the swings in a park, two miles down the road from the prison he was being released from that morning. In my rucksack, I had an envelope with £87 inside that one of my uncles had given me to pass on to Jason.

Jason showed up two hours late and smelling of weed. Seeing him made my heart break for how long it had been since I'd seen him. I handed him the envelope and we went to a pharmacy. The pharmacist gave Jason his daily prescription of methadone. It was 100ml – the highest dose possible. Jason turned his back to me and drank it.

We stepped out onto the street.

'Do you have to take methadone every day?' I asked.

'Yes. I never want you doing that,' he said.

'I'm not going to.'

'If you drank the prescription I just drank in there, it would kill you.'

I felt that being alive meant I owed a debt to my brother.

We walked into town. I was a big *Star Trek* fan at the time and could spend hours in front of my telly escaping into a world in which humanity had overcome all war, famine and disease. Jason offered to shoplift the complete series DVD boxset for me from a place in the arcade.

'You don't have to do that,' I said.

'I want to,' he said.

'I'm touched. But I don't want you to.'

'It might be difficult, anyway. I'm banned from the arcade.'

'Don't worry. It's the thought that counts.'

On the high street, Jason nodded to a friend of his, Chris, who was selling the *Big Issue*. 'Good to have you back, Jason,' Chris shouted. Two police officers saw this exchange. They came over and told Jason they were going to conduct a stop and search. Jason emptied his pockets and held out his arms. Chris complained they had no right to search Jason, then the officers searched Chris as well.

I took my phone, keys and wallet out of my pockets and stepped towards the officers.

'We don't need to search you,' one of them said.

I stood, holding out my things in my hand.

'Sir, please move away,' the officer said.

The fact that my life has been less punishing than Jason's has framed the way I experience almost everything. One of my favourite sensations is the excitement that comes in the moment the lights go down in the cinema and a film is about to start. When I was twenty, my brother went away for a year. I went to the cinema, the lights went down, but I didn't feel any anticipation. Instead, I felt nostalgic for how the experience had once been exciting. That pleasure had been lost to the fundamental problem: how could I be so lucky?

I didn't weep about Jason being away. Tears always felt imminent but never arrived. I'd feel stabs in my throat where I was almost welling up. Sadness, like excitement, was right there. But 'right there' was a world away.

During that period, I became preoccupied with TV shows and films about prison, like *Oz* and *Scum*. I watched them to keep some form of connection with Jason; trying not to look away at the violence on the screen. I read prison memoirs like John Healy's *The Grass Arena* and *In the Belly of the Beast* by Jack Henry Abbott; trying to understand how or if people survive dehumanization. I picked up Primo Levi's memoir about his imprisonment in Auschwitz *If This Is a Man*. It's about the most extreme forms of dehumanization that have ever taken place, so I was taken aback when I read the opening words 'It is my good fortune . . .'

Levi saw countless people marched to their execution but, by a cruel, arbitrary logic, he remained alive. It was his good fortune to have survived. Yet he was haunted by that luck; he couldn't shake the sense he was alive in another's place, as if he were 'his brother's Cain'. In the preface to *The Drowned and the Saved*, he said that he should not be considered a 'true witness' of Auschwitz. The only true witnesses, he thought, were those who had died. At the end of *The Truce*, he describes a recurring dream where he is sitting with friends in a garden. At first he feels serene, but a subtle anguish intrudes. Little by little, everything collapses and is destroyed, the scene, the walls, the people, until he's left alone at the centre of a grey murky void. Nothing outside the *Lager* is true.

Reading Levi's story challenged my ability to comprehend. The scale of it was far greater, and the structure more hellish, than my own story of being my brother's Cain. Nevertheless I felt grateful to Levi for showing so precisely how crushing survivor's shame can be to your sense of reality. One Sunday afternoon around that time, I was lying on my then-girlfriend Eleanor's sofa with my feet on her lap. She had been eating fruit and the room smelt of oranges. She started massaging the sole of my foot with her slim, elegant fingers. I closed my eyes to enjoy the feeling of relaxation. But a memory took hold in my mind.

The last time I'd seen Jason, we were sharing a hotel room together. Before bed, he needed to inject heroin so he could sleep. He poked the needle into the sole of his foot for about an hour before he found a vein. He kept saying sorry to me. He looked in so much pain.

Eleanor kept massaging my foot. I opened my eyes and looked at her hands squeeze my toes but I felt no release any more. It was like my foot was hollow inside. Eleanor pushed her hair behind her ear, but something about the movement seemed wrong, as if she were a puppet whose hand was being manipulated. She chatted to me, telling me things about her day, but it was as if her words had been broken down into separate sounds. I panicked that I didn't know how to put them back together again. I had the stark sense that everything was fake. I tried to say something back to Eleanor, but my words sounded tinny to me. I observed my voice passing out of my mouth.

I often had moments like that throughout my late teens and early twenties. I would be enjoying myself, think of Jason, and the force of his reality would make mine come apart. Wherever I was, I had to keep sight of my brother's suffering.

Jason hasn't been to prison since becoming a father, seven years ago. Today, he is happy, so I ought to be able to claim my happiness by extension. But working in prison, I meet people who are still in the throes of their ordeal. A month ago, I had a new student in my class who was a similar age to me called Reiss. He had a wide blond afro and several horizontal scars down his inner forearm. He told me that he wanted to get a tattoo to go over them, perhaps roses or cartoon characters or an entirely black sleeve.

Two weeks later, a prison guard came into my room before the class and handed me a red folder. It was a suicide watch document for Reiss. I opened it and saw entries made by officers the previous day: 'Ate some of his food.' 'Quiet.' 'Appeared tired.' At 2 a.m. the officer who looked through the inspection hatch of Reiss's cell wrote, 'In bed. Appeared to be breathing.' At 4 p.m. it read, 'Moved. Appeared to be alive.'

The following weekend, I was visiting a friend in the countryside and I went out running on the hills. I sprinted past my pain barrier. Endorphins were cascading in my brain. The sky was a limitless blue. The apple trees were abundant with white blossom. An image of Reiss in his cell was thrust into my mind. He was in his cell.

I came to a stop.

I looked out across the hills. They were a thing that Reiss couldn't see.

The day after my class with Patrick, I'm with my brother in his flat. He has two batik-style cushions on his sofa that he made at a support group for ex-drug users. They have stencilled blue elephants on them. Each time Jason stands up from the sofa, he fluffs the cushions and puts them back neatly. It's one of the lasting rituals of his recovery, along with washing up plates and cutlery the moment he's finished eating and checking every day to see if the fern on his windowsill needs water.

In my teens, Jason wasn't there, but I kept him at the front of my heart. Today, he stands in front of me. But I don't know what to do. Each time I go to his flat, I want to throw my arms around him, but instead I'm awkward, not sure where to stand or what to do with my hands. When Jason cleaned up, it was like he came back from the dead, but I wasn't done with my grief about him being gone. I needed him to tell me about the scars on his body, like how Saint Thomas wouldn't accept that Jesus had been resurrected until he touched Christ's wounds. But when my brother told me the story of how he got the scar on his thigh, I found it even harder to attach myself to the fact that he was alive.

Seven years on from when Jason painted the walls of his flat, the fact that he is here still seems only tentatively true. Sometimes I see the things in Jason's house – the cushions on the sofa, the plates and bowls and mugs, the TV and the coffee table – and imagine these objects might easily be put into a box and left out in the street. Strangers might come and pick through them and take things back to their homes. The absent Jason was the brother I grew up with. My love for him is as insistent as it ever was.

My brother now also has a two-year-old called Dean. On the sofa, Jason wants to show me a photo of his sons playing together in the park. He reaches for his pocket.

'Fucker,' he says.

Yesterday someone cycled past him on a bike and nicked his phone out of his hand.

A few minutes later, Jason wants to check a football score and reaches to his pocket again. 'Fuck. Bastard,' he says. 'My pictures, my contacts. I swear, Andy, I'm never nicking anyone's phone again.'

I burst out laughing.

Jason occasionally has these moments where he's the victim of a crime and he remembers how he has also been a perpetrator. One morning last year, he stepped out of the front door to find the windscreen of his girlfriend's car smashed in. He remembered a time fifteen years before when he broke into thirty or so cars in a single night. He'd forgotten about that until he was picking shards of glass off Dean's baby seat.

Twenty minutes later, Jason and I are in his kitchen. He's microwaving a vegetarian sausage roll he has bought especially for my visit.

'Are you still teaching in prison?' he asks.

'Yes,' I say.

'What was wrong with the job you had before?'

'I like this work.'

'I wish you'd be careful. Has anyone started on you?'

'They ask me how my holiday was with my boyfriend.'

'Why do you have to work in a prison?' he says.

When I was eighteen, Jason introduced me to one of his friends by saying, 'This is my little brother. He's never taken drugs or drank or even smoked a fag.' A few months later, that friend got high, fell asleep in the grass and didn't wake up. The following year Jason introduced me to another friend. 'Can you believe he's my brother? He's never touched anything.' That friend went to prison for four years. On the day he got out, he stole a car, crashed it into a wall and died. Today, when Jason introduces me to his mates, he still says, 'Andy has never done anything, no drugs or drink at all.' Jason doesn't like that I work in prison. He wants to keep my innocence alive.

In the kitchen, Jason reaches into his pocket for his phone. 'Bastards,' he says.

I laugh at him again.

'Which prison are you working in?' he asks.

'A high-security one. A couple of Victorian prisons. An open prison. I'm starting in a couple more next month,' I say.

The microwave pings. He opens it, takes out the plate and hands me my food.

'Fuck me, Bruv,' he says. 'You've almost been in as many prisons as me.'

Two days later, I'm walking to prison and I have a pain in one of my back teeth. I pass two pharmacies without going in to get some painkillers. Twenty minutes later, in prison, I step onto the wing. Five hundred men are being unlocked after fourteen hours banged up. I hear shouting, a rumble of footsteps and alarms from a cell on the landing above me. Adrenaline fizzes through my limbs and I no longer feel the pain in my tooth.

A few minutes later, I set up the circle of chairs in my class, minus one seat because Osman isn't coming any more. I have the red folder for Reiss on my desk. The room is bathed in grey light coming through the window that faces onto the prison wall. An officer outside shouts, 'Free flow.'

Barry is the first to arrive, a Welshman with a finger

missing on his right hand. He has previously told me he's in because of a joke that his friend didn't find funny. He has a shrill laugh. It cuts through me; my tooth throbs again.

Reiss comes in and takes a seat. He's wearing a fresh white T-shirt and looks dazed. Not sleepy, but just absent, as if he is slightly stoned or has just changed his medication. The rest of the men trickle in and take a seat. The two men on either side of Reiss talk to each other, but Reiss aloofly stares at his nails.

I close the door and get the class underway.

I say, 'The Roman politician Boethius is in a prison cell. Lady Philosophy appears to him.'

'A female comes in his cell?' Barry asks.

'Boethius is imagining her. She's a literary device. He's lamenting his bad luck for being jailed. Lady Philosophy gives him a teaching.'

'I might have met Lady Philosophy when I was lamenting in my cell,' says Barry.

A few men snicker. My tooth aches.

Barry says, 'What had he been nicked for?'

'Treason,' I say. 'Though all he really did was stay loyal to the old regime during a change of power. While he waits to be executed, he cries, "Fortune should feel ashamed for punishing an innocent man." So, Lady Philosophy teaches him what Fortuna, the Roman goddess of luck, is really like.'

'There's a lady and a goddess in his cell?' Barry says.

'We don't even get conjugal visits,' Jerome says. Jerome is in his early fifties and has been in and out of jail since he was a teenager. His accent shifts back and forth between the Irish of his childhood and the cockney of his life now. He has thick grey arms. I cannot see any veins under his skin, from where they have died. He knew the governor in this prison when she was an officer in training. He has a boyish smile and a trembling hand.

I say, 'Lady Philosophy tells Boethius that he is actually lucky.'

'Yes,' Jerome says. 'Just because you're locked up doesn't mean you're not lucky.'

The men grunt in agreement. One man mutters that he's lucky that his mother still visits him. Another mentions he has a radio. Talk ripples through the room. They talk about how they are lucky: having a single cell, surviving a stabbing, a job mopping the landing. 'Being in here safeguards the people I love,' Reiss says.

I feel a throb of pain in my back tooth. I cup my face with my hand and close my eyes.

'Got a sore tooth? Go to healthcare!' Barry says.

I take my hand away from my face. 'It's nothing.'

'Ask the dentist to give you something. Or if you ask around on the wing, you could get something a bit stronger,' Barry says.

Barry laughs at his own joke. I massage my gum with my tongue to try to ease the pain.

'Can you take me with you?' Barry continues. 'I've been trying to get them to see me for months. Every time my appointment comes round, there's a lockdown and I can't go.'

'You'll get an abscess,' I say.

'The pain is just normal now,' Barry says.

'I just have overly sensitive teeth,' I say.

'How do you know? You've got to look after yourself, Andy.'

★

A few moments later, Reiss takes the lid off the top of his pen, puts it between his front teeth and bites it. He moves the lid over to his back teeth and crunches down. I hear the plastic crack.

I say, 'Lady Philosophy tells Boethius that he is actually lucky. She reminds him that he has a father-in-law who feels angry about Boethius's suffering, a wife who still loves him and children who behave well. Lady Philosophy tells him, "Nothing is wretched, only thinking makes it so."'

'Luck is all a matter of perception,' Jerome says. 'No matter how bad your situation is, you can still think of yourself as lucky. My cellmate is from Eritrea. He can't believe how nice it is in here. He says that in his country they shut prisoners up in shipping containers in the middle of the desert, thirty at a time. I hear that and it puts things in perspective.'

'But a man who sees every situation as lucky is delusional,' Barry says.

'Or he hasn't lost his imagination yet,' Jerome says.

'I've got a cellmate who never says anything all day and laughs all night in his sleep,' Barry says.

'You can find positives in that,' Jerome says.

'Come back and tell me that when you're as sleep-deprived as I am,' Barry says.

Jerome's hand is trembling. 'I'm not saying being positive is always a good thing.'

I lean forward and ask, 'Why not?'

'It's really easy to feel lucky in prison,' Jerome says. 'I can look around and in two seconds see someone worse off than me. You didn't know your dad; he didn't know his dad or his mum. You was adopted; the next bloke never went to school. Thinking I was lucky has helped me bounce back. But being good at bouncing back isn't something I feel that proud of any more. Because I know I can bounce back from messy situations, I stop caring about if I get into messy situations or not.'

'Does that mean you should stop thinking that you're lucky?' I ask.

'I'm not the type to call myself unlucky. But I can't keep calling myself lucky either. I need another word,' Jerome says.

'What would that word be?' I ask.

I hear the sound of keys in the door. A guard opens it. Osman comes in, the man who left my class to take a job in the kitchen. He collects a chair from the edge of the room and sits in the circle. The officer closes the door and locks it behind him.

I say, 'I thought you—'

'I don't wanna talk about it,' he says.

'OK. We're talking about Fortuna, the Roman goddess of lu—'

'My fucking brother!' Osman says. 'My mum didn't tell me he was in here. That's not a surprise – she thinks he can do no wrong.'

'What happened?' Jerome says.

'I've been working in the kitchen for the last few days. Working so flat out. It's been great. I've been sleeping like a baby. Then I walk in today and he's in there, my little brother. He's blagged himself a job in the kitchen.'

'Don't give up a kitchen job, Osman. Just try and forget he's there,' Jerome says.

'He hates cooking and washing up. He's only took that job to wind me up,' Osman says.

The men look at each other and make awkward faces.

Osman rests his elbows on his knees and massages his temples with his thumbs.

A few minutes later, Jerome and Barry debate Lady Philosophy's idea that 'Nothing is wretched, only thinking makes it so.'

Barry puts his hand in the air and says, 'Happy people tend to say they're lucky, don't they? Boethius is trying to reverse-engineer a bit of happiness by telling himself he's lucky. It's like Lady Philosophy has given him permission to print money. But we all know he's not actually lucky. He's just dreamed up a woman telling him he is so he doesn't blow his own fucking brains out.'

I look at Reiss. He moves the pen lid from one side of his mouth to the other using his tongue. He sucks the saliva back, swallows and keeps chewing.

Jerome leans forward and says, 'But Boethius has been unfairly banged up. Got eleven months for something I didn't do once. I've done lots of prison. I did six years and seven months once and I deserved every day of it because I was guilty. But the eleven months was harder to get through than the six years.'

'Why?' I ask.

Jerome says, 'On the six, I was positive. I was reading, going to the gym, support groups, helping people out who'd just come to prison. But on the eleven months, the only energy I could find was rage. I couldn't get over how unfair it was. It was like I punched my way through every single day of that sentence.'

'Does that mean Boethius thinks of himself as lucky?' I ask.

'If he doesn't he'll burn himself out,' Jerome says.

My tooth throbs again. I look around the group. Osman looks like he doesn't want anyone to talk to him. Reiss's eyelids are lowered, so I can't make out his mood. I ask him, 'Does Boethius have to think he's lucky?'

Reiss takes the pen lid out of his mouth. The black plastic is gnarled with teeth marks. He sucks in the excess saliva. 'How long was Boethius in for?' Reiss says.

'Only until his execution. Not long,' I say.

'Would Lady Philosophy still be telling Boethius he's lucky if she was visiting him after ten years?' Reiss asks.

'I don't know. Should she?' I say.

Reiss shrugs.

I say, 'The German philosopher Hegel thought Boethius's attitude did strange things to people over time.'

I see a flicker of emotion in Reiss's face. 'Like what?'

'Hegel said that if you kept repeating a mantra about how nothing in the world is actually bad, but only your thinking makes it bad, then over time, you'll lose connection with the world. The universe becomes no bigger than our own skull. We become detached, alienated and unhappy.'

'Boethius is never going back into the world,' Reiss says. 'He's gonna die inside anyway.'

Barry says, 'What Hegel's saying is that Boethius has to stop spending so much time with imaginary women. Otherwise, if he's ever faced with an actual naked woman, he won't know what to do with her.'

Barry laughs at his own joke. Reiss puts the pen lid back in his mouth and keeps crunching on it.

Twenty minutes later, a security officer in the corridor outside shouts, 'Free flow' to signal it's time for the men to go back to their cells. My students file towards the door. Barry pats me on the arm and tells me to make sure I get to the dentist. Osman lingers behind. 'I'm sorry about earlier, Andy. It's just my fucking brother.'

'Family can be—'

'I had my head down. I was happy doing my time. Now he's in here. To be honest with you, I just want to get out of prison now.'

Osman leaves and I close the door behind him. I go to my desk, open the red folder where I have to record how Reiss was today. I flick forward to an unmarked page and note down that Reiss looked a bit woozy, but he contributed, mostly followed what was going on, laughed at some points but not at others.

I feel another throb of pain in my tooth. I look at what I've written. I can't see how anything I've put is meaningful. I add something else, saying he was relaxed but not worryingly calm. But that doesn't seem much better. I massage my gum with my tongue. I add that he didn't seem aggressive and got on with the others, but I just feel like I'm multiplying empty statements.

A few minutes later, an officer with ginger hair comes into my room. 'We're trying to locate a red folder, sir?'

'I won't be long,' I say.

He walks up behind me and looks over my shoulder. 'You've put enough there for a suicide report. What happened?'

'He was OK today.'

The officer takes the folder off the desk and puts it under his arm. 'It's lunch. Go outside.'

Happiness

> It was the very discomfort, the blows, the cold,
> the thirst that kept us aloft in the void of
> bottomless despair.
>
> Primo Levi

Before I could start working in prison, I had to fill out numerous security clearance forms. One document asked, 'Do you have any relatives imprisoned? Please tick Yes or No.' Next to the 'No' box I wrote: 'Not at the moment.'

Two years ago, Mum messaged me to say my uncle Frank had just got out after doing three years inside. He was staying at my nan's council flat in the East End of London. The last time I'd seen my uncle was ten years before, at a family wedding. He was wearing a £2,000 Armani suit. I needed a new computer at the time and Frank told me he had recently acquired 300 laptops, but sadly none of them had any innards.

I took the bus to my nan's flat. The concrete stairwell on her block smelt of urine. Opposite her building was a house with St George's flags hanging out of all four windows. Next to the house was an Evangelical church. It had red bricks and double-glazed windows. A group of women with what sounded like Nigerian accents were talking in the doorway.

I knocked at my nan's door and Frank opened. His face looked rounder than it had done at the wedding, thanks to three years of regular meals in prison.

'You look well, Unc,' I said.

He slapped his belly. 'I'm turning into a fat fucker. Hope I can keep it up,' he said.

Frank took me into the kitchen and made us both tea. He put three sugars in his and asked me how many I have. 'None,' I said. He rolled a cigarette, tearing off a corner from an old lottery ticket and using it as a roach. 'Do you want a fag?' he asked.

'I don't smoke,' I said.

We went into the living room. On the wall, there was a faded picture of Marilyn Monroe which Nan had had for forty years. The pale green carpet was fluffy from where Nan hoovered every other day. I sat in an armchair and Frank sat on the arm of the sofa. Through the window, I could see Canary Wharf. Nan watched daytime cooking programmes. Her false teeth were in a jar on the coffee table.

Frank didn't have his false teeth in either. He sucked on his cigarette and told me about the time he was in an exercise yard during a previous stint in a low-security prison eight or nine years ago.

'The day was baking. Me and Vinnie had the volleyball court to just us,' he said.

I leaned forward, straining to try to hear him over the sound of the TV.

He said, 'We was only supposed to get an hour but the screws was giving us more. The screws had their collars undone, we was all getting a bit of sun.'

Nan sighed. Frank loved telling jail stories and she hated hearing them. She took her false teeth out of the jar on the coffee table and put them in her mouth. That was her way of rising above it.

'We're bouncing this ball to each other, and then . . .'

Frank edged to the corner of the sofa and drew his hands apart, 'there's this bees' nest on the wall. It's been there the last few days apparently. Everyone was staying well away. So, Vinnie gives me a look. But I reckon we should keep playing for a bit first cos the day was so nice.'

My nan picked up the remote and turned up the volume on a shopping channel. It was showcasing anti-ageing eyeshadow.

'The screws were about to call time, rounding everyone up. Vinnie sees the screw put the whistle to his mouth and kicks the ball at the nest. You should have seen it, Andy. The sky went black. Bees fucking everywhere.'

Nan switched off the TV, groaned and shuffled out of the room.

'They nicked us for that,' he said. 'Three more days inside, we had to do. They didn't know what to charge us with, so they just put "aggravating bees" on the bit of paper.'

'Why did you do it?' I asked.

'How do you mean?'

'Why did you hit the bees' nest?'

'Because it made an already sweet day even sweeter.'

When Frank was fourteen years old, he stole a crate of Coca-Cola from a shop in the East End. He was arrested and held in prison on remand for four months. When his case finally went to court, the judge said it was appalling to have held a child of Frank's age in custody for that length of time and dismissed the case. Frank returned to prison in less than a year for theft. He went on to become a professional burglar. He has never done people's homes, and he has refused offers to join armed robberies because, in his words, 'The bird is just too long.' Warehouses and department store stockrooms were his trade.

When Frank got out two years ago, he found most of his mates were now either dead, doing seriously long sentences or just too old for the game. Vinnie had become a Hare Krishna, only to then be arrested for a crime he'd committed before his conversion. Inside, the other men laughed at Vinnie for the prayer beads he wore around his wrist. During association, he wore a carrier bag over his right hand to hide his beads. Vinnie hasn't wanted to go back to prison since.

I saw my uncle Frank half a dozen times the summer he got out. He knew I was curious about him and took that as provocation to launch into storytelling at any moment when we were together. One midweek afternoon, I was with Frank at my nan's house. He was telling me about a time thirty years ago when he and Vinnie had to serve a two-year sentence in HMP Canterbury.

'On day one, they hated us. They were shouting "You fucking London cunts" as we walked down the landing. I looked at Vinnie and said, "We're gonna get killed in here." On the second day, in the shower, two blokes walked in. I knew they would, so I'd brought a bit of wood in with me that I'd ripped off a table. One of their blokes had a battery in a sock.'

'Where were security?' I said.

'They'd turned a blind eye, Andy.'

'Why?'

'What you gotta remember, Andy, is these were the days when screws wore National Front badges on their uniform. Anyway, the geezer comes in with a battery in a sock, but it was a long sock and he was holding it at the top, so it hung about a foot long. I saw that and I knew they didn't know what they were doing. You're supposed to hold it just a few inches from the battery, so as soon as the bloke swings it at Vinnie, I grab the middle of the sock so the geezer can't use it. Then Vinnie hit the fuckers with the wood until one of their heads starts bleeding, and they all run off.'

'Did that come back on you?' I asked.

'We used to have a puff with those blokes in the end. Canterbury was wonderful because it was right near Dover where the lorries came off the ferry. I tried drugs in that prison that I didn't even know existed – Blonde Lebanese, Red Moroccan, Afghani Fingers. After two years, me and Vinnie had to leave because we'd served our time. We didn't want to go.'

'But you were always on downers, right? You wanted to swallow the days.'

'We did LSD in our cell. The guards told us to keep it down because we were laughing so loud all night. All the experiences I've had – I've met every type of person there is in prison, every type of drug. I don't regret anything.'

I scanned his face for any emotion that might contradict the words coming from his mouth. I couldn't tell if he really believed it or not.

'What about when you got nicked?' I said. 'Didn't you feel regret then?'

'The time we got nicked before last, the police was asking us if we wanted milk and sugar in our tea, calling us sir and checking if there was anything they could do for us. They was as good as gold. A lot of these coppers are normally just scraping around picking up two-bob criminals, shoplifters and junkies. But we was professionals. They'd been trying to catch us for two years. They had a map of England on the wall with pins in it for all of the work we'd done.'

After the Berlin Wall came down, some East Berliners experienced 'the wall in the head' – the feeling that they still couldn't travel to the other side of the city. Some people get released from prison and feel a similar sense of residual confinement. They are out, but in their head they are still inside. During the conversations I had with my uncle last summer, I kept interrupting his stories to ask questions like 'How come you did that?' or 'But didn't you get in trouble for that?' Frank had to go back to explain the ABC of it to me. When he cracked a punchline, my laughter often lagged behind. I wasn't sure when he was joking and when he was being serious. I went back and forth between feeling incredulous and ignorant. I felt like I experienced the wall in the head but from the other side. I couldn't get in.

This aggravated a long-standing wound. I'd lost my brother to prison and although I felt relief when my dad went away, I still missed having a dad. Men had so often been out of reach for me. With my uncle, I was experiencing that separation again.

Today, I'm in a Victorian jail. It is five landings tall and has single wings that hold more men than some entire prisons do. I walk down the second-floor landing, or 'the twos' as it's called, towards my classroom. A man shouts through the inspection hatch of his cell door. His rant is directed at the officers. 'This ain't fair. I'm gonna fuck you up!' he says. His yelling is lost in the cacophony of other men shouting and banging from behind their cell doors.

I slow my walk to glance inside the cells where a door is open. In one, I see a middle-aged man in tracksuit bottoms. He's sat on his bed watching telly, drinking a mug of tea and smoking a vape. My uncle has jailed in this prison a few times over the decades. One of these cells would have been his.

I go up the metal staircase to the third floor. A young man slouching against the railings outside his cell says, 'Miss, this is bullshit.' He's wearing a vest and has the words NO REGRETS tattooed across his collarbone. A female officer comes out of his cell carrying a TV. If men break the rules, the officers can put them on 'basic', meaning the prison reduces the length of the prisoner's visits, how much money they are able to earn, and takes away their TV.

The officer carries his TV away towards the office.

'Fuck, what do I care anyway. I'll just get another one.'

Sometimes when people get put on basic, they nick a telly from another cell.

I need the loo, but I won't make it to the staff toilet and back in time for the start of my class. Instead, I head to the single cubicle in the education corridor, which both students and teachers can use. The door is covered in graffiti and has a large square hole where the glass has been removed. I push it open and go inside. The stench of stale piss is so strong I have to hold my breath so as not to retch. The sink is coming apart from the wall. Vertical copper-coloured streaks are so encrusted onto the porcelain of the toilet they look like they have been engraved into it. The U-bend is black with decay. There is a film on the surface of the water that shimmers indigo and green.

I urinate. I press the lever using only the tip of my finger. The water flushes. It makes the smell of stale piss even stronger. I hold my nose and hurry out of the toilet.

A few minutes later, I'm in my classroom. I take my books for today's class out of my bag and onto the desk. I set up the chairs in a circle. I glance up at the wall, where the clock normally is, but it's been taken away. I'm not wearing a watch. I put my head out of the door and see a security officer walking down the corridor.

I say, 'Excuse me, is there a clock in one of the other rooms I could borrow, please?'

The officer steps into my classroom. He's about sixty, wiry and has a splotchy tattoo of a mermaid on his forearm. His ID badge shows his name – Adamson. He looks me up and down.

'I should've brought my watch,' I say.

'Things go missing for a reason here. A CD went missing from a classroom last month. A prisoner had snapped it to make a shank.'

'They'd attack each other with clocks?' I ask.

'It's good to have your own watch in this place.'

'Fair enough. I just thought I'd ask.'

'You'd be amazed what they can make into a weapon. These men have a lot of time on their hands for new inventions.'

Adamson speaks with the same old-fashioned East London accent as my uncle. 'They'll snap a toilet brush to make a shank. Make sure they don't take any of your pens when they leave. I've seen what they can do to someone's neck.'

I have to get ready for my class. Normally officers don't

talk to me for this long. They often respond to me tersely, like I'm distracting them from something. But Adamson is listing off the reasons why I can't have a clock. I nod my head and say 'Understood', 'Yes' and 'I bet', in the hope that it will hurry him along to the end of his spiel and he will leave.

'They can take the batteries out of a clock, put them in a sock and then whack someone over the head with it,' he says.

I walk over to the computer and tap the mouse to activate the screen.

'There's the time on here, look,' I say.

Adamson carries on. 'Then we'll have an incident.'

I point to the corner of the screen. 'Is that the time already?'

'And an incident means paperwork.'

I clench my jaw shut, hoping that if I stop saying things, then he might stop saying things too.

'What do you do here, then?' he says.

'I'm a philosophy teacher,' I say.

'So, what do you *do* here, then?'

He looks down at the pile of philosophy books on my desk. He taps his finger on one called *The Philosophy of Happiness*. I feel embarrassed, like a teenager who has just been caught doing something shameful by a grandparent.

'A lot of them in here are happy to be in prison.' He shakes his head. 'And I thought prison was supposed to be hard.'

An officer in the corridor shouts 'Free flow' and Adamson turns and leaves.

A man called Jim is the first student to arrive. A former

SAS soldier, he has a broad chest and strong arms. He gives me his usual shoulder-bump greeting. I hold my stomach in.

'Good morning,' I say.

He sighs and looks around the room. Jim is as emotionally weary as he is physically strong. His ears are covered with tufts of auburn hair, as if to block out the sound of the landing.

A new student walks in, who introduces himself as Salvatore. He has bright blue eyes and the word 'Cheers' is on the front of his T-shirt, from the American TV series. He gives me an elaborate handshake which I can't keep up with. He tries again and talks me through the choreography of stages; the clasp, the clicking together of thumbs, the wriggling of fingers and the high five. 'Good morning, brother,' he says.

'How are you?' I ask.

'I'm OK,' he says. He puts his hand over his heart. 'I'm always OK, brother,' he says. He turns to shake Jim's hand, but Jim keeps his arms folded. Salvatore puts his hand over his heart. 'Namaste,' he says.

Salvatore looks a little over twenty-five. He tells me he's twenty-two days into a nine-month sentence. This is his first time inside.

'Sorry to hear that,' I say.

'Why are you sorry?' he says. 'I've accepted it. Time is moving fast for me because I'm not resisting the truth. I'm in here. This is where I'm meant to be. I'm not gonna let it make me miserable. This is a learning experience. I'm learning from this. Don't be sorry for me, brother. I've accepted it. Now it's time to give something back. I've told my cellmate that I'm gonna teach him lizard lunge – a yoga pose that makes you accept what is there. The sooner we accept what's happening to us, the quicker the time passes. Time is a me—'

'Can we just get on with the lesson?' Jim says.

Jim is a third of the way through a fourteen-year sentence. He takes a seat on the other side of the circle from Salvatore.

Half a dozen other men arrive. A twenty-one-year-old called Yusuf comes in and sits at a table with his back to the circle. I go over to check if he's OK. He's filling out an application to request that he be moved to a single cell. He explains that last week an officer asked him if he wanted a cellmate who was also a Muslim like him. Yusuf said yes.

'But I can't live with this bloke,' Yusuf says. 'He threw away all my chocolate biscuits because he said they weren't halal. The other night I'm watching a film and twenty minutes in a woman in a short skirt comes on and he changes the channel. He said cos it's not pious to watch it. He does that every time he sees a woman's legs on the screen. Or even a shoulder. A shoulder for fuck's sake!'

'Do your application. Join us when you're ready,' I say.

'The guvs best move me. I need a single cell. I can't live like this.'

I go to the door and close it. On the whiteboard, I write 'Bentham' and 'Happiness = Pleasure'. I say, 'The philosopher Jeremy Bentham defin—'

The classroom door opens and Adamson steps inside. He's holding a white wall clock. He rests it upright against a computer.

Puzzled, I point at the computer screen behind me. 'I can just use—'

Adamson steps out of the door and closes it behind him.

The class look at me, waiting for me to carry on.

I say, 'Bentham thought that happiness and pleasure were the same thing. When I say I'm happy, I'm experiencing pleasure. When I say I'm feeling pleasure, I'm happy.'

'You can be happy in prison, did you know that?' Salvatore says.

Yusuf turns around and looks at Salvatore as if he's about to shoot laser beams out of his eyes.

'I still feel pleasure, every day, even though I'm in here. I had my coffee this morning and I made sure to really enjoy it. I wasn't complaining that it wasn't gourmet. Once you accept you're in here, you can enjoy those pleasures again.'

Jim looks more tired with each word that comes out of Salvatore's mouth.

Salvatore goes on. 'I hear people tell me they're bored. Do you know what they mean by that? I don't. I've never been bored in my life. There's no cell in my mind. People say to me, "Salvatore, why do you always smile so much?" and I tell them—'

'He designed prisons,' Jim interrupts, pointing at the name 'Jeremy Bentham' on the board. 'He was the one who designed the panopticon.'

'The what?' Salvatore asks.

'I thought you knew everything about prison,' Jim says.

Salvatore gives Jim a priestly smile.

'Bentham designed the Millbank prison,' Jim says. 'It was a circle shape with a viewing spot in the middle. The screws could see you, but you couldn't see them, so you never knew if the screws were watching you or not. This place is based on there.'

'So, if Bentham designed places like this, do you think he knows what happiness is?' I ask.

'I don't know. I stopped thinking about him the moment I realized who he was,' Jim says.

'Come on, brother. Did you know it uses twice as many muscles to frown as it does to smile,' says Salvatore.

'How many does it take to keep your mouth shut?' Jim says.

Two nights later, I'm in my nan's living room, sat next to Frank. The fire is on and the windows closed. The faint smell of battered fish lingers in the air from dinner time. On the coffee table, my nan has set down a plate of Penguin chocolate bars, a dozen chocolate biscuits and three chocolate eclairs.

The fact that I now work in prisons Frank takes as further provocation to launch into telling stories about his time inside without warning. Since I've been working in jails, there's been a change in the way I hear his stories. It's as if there's more space around his words. He mentions the wing and it's as if I can walk around it. I can hear the din of the landing and smell the stale air.

I tell Frank that I've started teaching in a prison he used to be in.

'Can you remember the number of your cell?' I ask.

'I can remember the exercise yard was an old graveyard,' he says. 'It was full of the bodies of prisoners they'd hung over the years.'

He closes one eye to think.

He says, 'Vinnie always got sulky with me in there because my shits smelt so bad. In them days you just shat in a bucket. I used to wrap mine in newspaper and throw it out the window. Loads of people did that. The whole yard was full of shit parcels. If the screws didn't like you, then they'd send you out to pick them all up.'

'Do you remember what wing you were on?' I ask.

'Nah. I was probably only there two or three times, if I'm honest,' he says.

The air in the living room is warm and stuffy. I nudge Frank and say, 'The weather is supposed to be good next week. We could go to the heath?'

'If you like,' he shrugs. 'Fancy you working in the same prison I was in. What's it like there now?'

'Quite rowdy at the moment,' I say.

Frank's face lights up.

'People are irritable since the smoking ban,' I say.

'The what?'

'They banned smoking in all prisons last year. Even in the yard.'

'Oh my god.'

'Tobacco is illegal inside. People vape now.'

'They've done what? That's it. I'm never going to prison again now. How dare they.'

When Frank was a kid, he'd jump on the train without a ticket and evade the conductor until the train got to Sandwich in Kent. He'd go to the nature reserves along the coast, sit on the shore and watch the sun go down.

Frank makes us our sixth cup of tea of the afternoon, comes back into the living room and hands it to me. I blow the steam away from my tea. He sits on the arm of the sofa next to me, his elbow touching my shoulder. I smell cigarette smoke on his clothes. Outside the window, the sun is glinting off Canary Wharf.

I nudge Frank again and say, 'We could go to Sandwich?'

'I used to go egging there as a kid.'

'Egging?'

'Robbing birds' eggs. I used to collect them. I had a turquoise-green crow egg. A speckled brown one what came from a kestrel. You can't do it now though. There's too much security.'

'Why don't we go to Sandwich? We can get some fresh air together,' I say.

'All right, let's go when we have a clear day. On a clear day, you can see tons of different birds in the sky and in the trees. You can see kingfishers, cuckoos, ospreys.'

'The weather isn't bad now,' I say.

'Yeah, let's wait for a clear day,' he says.

A moment later, Frank tells me about when he was fifteen years old and spent six months in a borstal, which used to be famous for its Short Sharp Shock regime. I set my mug down on the coffee table to let it cool.

'At feeding, you had to stand to attention outside your cell, they'd call your name, you was supposed to march down,' he says.

He stands up from the arm of the sofa, tightens his mouth into a face of seriousness and marches a few steps across the living room with slapstick exaggeration.

'But I just went down like this,' he said.

He turns and does the most extravagant swagger for a few steps, scuffing his feet, leaving trail marks in the fluffy carpet.

He sits back on the arm of the sofa and says, 'The screw punched me in the stomach for that. But the next day I did it again, not marching. I did that every day. Every day they punched me in the stomach.'

His face turns to a grin.

'Then the screws changed tack. They called out my name. I strolled down and they gave me my dinner, but they'd covered my whole plate in salt. I had to scrape it all off with my knife. But every day I kept on not marching. They kept on handing me a plate of food that was white with salt. After a week of that they threw me in the seg.'

The seg is the segregation unit.

I pick my mug up from the coffee table and wrap both my hands around it.

He says, 'Down there you're just sleeping on a concrete ledge. The screws would wake me up every morning and take me outside and give me a shovel and make me dig a hole eight foot deep. It's all fucking wet and clay down there. Then at the end of the day, I'd have to fill the hole back in. The next morning, they'd wake me up and take me outside and make me do the same again. Digging holes and filling them back in again.'

'Didn't you end up swinging a shovel at someone's head? You must have gone mad,' I say.

'When the screw opened my door in the morning, I'd spring to my feet and give him a big smile. I'd say, "I love digging holes."'

'But you hated it?' I say.

'I just used to pretend I loved it. I loved it.'

I feel like I am on the other side of the wall to him again. I set my mug down on the table and turn my neck to look Frank directly in the eyes.

'But you didn't love it, did you?' I say.

He stands up from the arm of the sofa, takes a roll-up cigarette from behind his ear and puts it in his mouth. 'I loved it, Andy. I just used to pretend I loved it.'

A couple of days later, I'm in a high-security prison. In the teachers' staffroom, the cookery teacher tells me that a security issue two days ago has meant the class temporarily cannot use any knives, hot water and most kitchen utensils, in case they get smuggled back on the wing and used as weapons. The cookery teacher is also not allowed to bring in food, as security are trying to crack down on staff smuggling in drugs. She told me how, this morning, she mimed to the men how to cut an onion, with no knife or onion; how the knuckles should be in front of the fingertips so the men didn't cut themselves. The men mimed this action and she corrected them where necessary. One man pretended to cry from the onion fumes.

The following morning, in the Victorian prison, I walk past the horrible toilet, catching the smell of stale piss. I go into my classroom and the whiteboard is full of notes from an anger-management class held last week. The words 'Respect', 'Escalation' and 'Rage' are written in capitals with red arrows going between them. I take the board rubber to wipe them out, but it has no effect. I rub harder, but the words won't come off. Whoever wrote them on used a permanent marker.

I stick my head out of the corridor and see Officer Adamson. I flag him down and he walks towards me. He holds a supermarket BLT sandwich and a packet of Haribo fizzy sweets.

'There wouldn't be a whiteboard spray anywhere, would there?' I say.

'Any liquids like that have to come into the prison sealed if you want to bring them in,' he says.

'I'll try hot soapy water.'

He looks at me like I am an extraterrestrial. 'You want to carry hot water through the building?'

'My whiteboard is covered in someone else's lesson. Can I get another one from somewhere?'

'If I go and start rummaging around for a whiteboard for your psychology class and I'm out of position here—'

'I'll just make notes on paper instead.'

'And if I'm out of position when something kicks off—'

His radio sounds, and he lifts the receiver closer to his ear. I use this as an opportunity to get away. I go back into my classroom and shut the door.

I get an A4 piece of paper and draw a man pushing a giant boulder up a mountain. I place the sheet in the middle of the circle of chairs.

The officer in the corridor shouts, 'Free flow.' A man called Gurman is the first to arrive. He's in his mid-twenties and used to be an outdoor activities instructor before coming to prison. He is freshly shaved and full of energy. Ten minutes later, nobody else has arrived, because the biggest wing in the prison hasn't been unlocked yet because of an incident.

'Can't we just start anyway?' Gurman says.

'I'd just have to explain everything all over again when the others get here,' I say.

'We are going to be waiting ages,' he says. He goes to the table at the back of the room where magazines and newspapers are kept and looks for the most recent newspaper. He finds it. It's two weeks old. He flicks through four or five pages and drops it back on the table.

A couple of months ago, Gurman asked his mum to send him a clock for his cell. The one she sent had a second hand that didn't tick but moved smoothly and continuously. Gurman said he found it 'relentless'. A few days later, he swapped it for a packet of biscuits.

Ten minutes later, Jim arrives. 'Some idiot threw a cup of piss at a screw,' he says. 'Meanwhile we have to wait to be unlocked while they carted him off to the seg and cleaned up the mess. I'm sick of these fucking heroes fucking up my morning.'

Salvatore trails into the room. His blue eyes look red and raw. He sits down in the chair next to Jim. Jim doesn't look happy about it.

Everyone is here. I sit in the circle of chairs. I point to the drawing on the floor in the middle. 'This is Sisyphus. He—'

'They've taken my cellmate away,' Salvatore says. 'They've put him in the seg. Now I'm alone in my cell.'

'What you complaining about? I'd love a cell to myself,' Jim says.

'He used to kill the cockroaches,' Salvatore says. 'Last night, I kept thinking I could feel them crawling on me. I didn't sleep at all last night. The bastards are everywhere.'

A man standing behind Salvatore tickles Salvatore's ear. Salvatore slaps his hand away and says, 'Please.' His voice sounds like he's on the edge of tears. 'I can't believe I've got another eight months in this place. Eight months!'

'Do you think you might try and be a bit more sensitive,'

Jim says. 'Some of us are doing tens and twenties. How do you think it makes me feel to hear you complaining that you got eight months?'

Four or five other men grunt in agreement. 'I was only out nine days before I got recalled here,' one says. Another says, 'It's three hours here, three hours back on the train for my kids to visit me down here. Do you know how much that costs?'

Salvatore says, 'I'm sorry. I shouldn't complain, but—'

'I never said you shouldn't complain,' Jim says.

Salvatore's face softens. He looks heartened by Jim's words. 'We're all in this together, I know. It's just someti—'

'You can complain all you like,' Jim says. 'Just don't complain to me. I wake up happy every day here. And I'll do the same tomorrow and the next day. I'm not going to let anyone spoil it.'

Salvatore's face crumples in despair. 'Why don't they put another cellmate in with me? I thought this bloody place was supposed to be overcrowded.'

'I thought you'd come in here to give something back,' Jim says, a smile forming in the corner of his mouth.

Salvatore's shoulders are slumped. His face looks ashen. He's quiet, no longer churning out self-help slogans. It's dawning on him that he's in prison. I get up from my chair and go to the corner of the room where I keep bottles of tap water and plastic cups. I pour a drink of water, pass it to Salvatore and take my seat. Salvatore puts the cup on the floor beside his chair leg.

Sat next to Salvatore is a twenty-one-year-old man called Amir. He has two lion tattoos, one on both forearms. 'You've gotta make the most of your time in here,' he says. He holds his fists up to his face like a boxer. 'Prison is my training.'

'Is there boxing here?' Salvatore asks.

Everyone laughs at him.

'Prison is the ring,' Amir says. 'I follow Floyd Mayweather's three principles. Keep your distance. Use your jab. Avoid a brawl.'

Salvatore looks puzzled.

'Keep your distance: I only listen to someone for fifteen seconds. If their conversation is negative, I'm gone. Use your jab: I get in and then get out. I get my food and take it back to my cell. I shower and then I go back to my cell. I don't drift around on the landing mixing with people. I keep myself to myself. This is not the time or place for friends. Avoid a brawl: I don't get caught up in nonsense. People use fighting in here as entertainment, but it's draining. I don't want to be a thug. I'm a warrior.'

'Thank you, brother,' Salvatore says. 'Do you think the officers will give me a new cellmate before tonight?'

'I don't think anything. I keep my distance, I use my jab and I don't get into brawls.'

Salvatore blinks. Worry etches itself deeper into his face.

I sit in the circle with Salvatore, Jim, Gurman, Amir and the others. I point to the drawing on the floor of a man pushing a boulder up a mountain. 'This is Sisyphus,' I say. 'In the underworld, the gods made him push a boulder up a mountain. When he pushed it to the top, it would roll back down. He would have to head down the mountain and push it all the way up again. When he got to the top, the giant rock would roll back down.'

The men laugh. Salvatore's expression is becoming ever more grave.

'He had to go back down the mountain and push the boulder to the top where it would roll back down, and then he'd have to go back down and push it to the top, over and over again.'

'We had to do something like that, but with bins,' Brendan says. Brendan is seventy-three. His voice has the creaky nasal sound that comes from years of intense drug use. 'They put me in military prison when I was sixteen for desertion.' He sucks in a breath between sentences. 'They gave us this big black dustbin and I had to sand all the black paint off it to take it back to the steel, and then buff the steel and bring it up so you could see your face in it.' He sucks in another breath. 'When the screw was happy with it, they'd give us a pot of black paint and you'd have to paint it again.'

'I'd prefer to be doing that,' Gurman says. 'I thought I was actually going to be punished by coming to jail, but I just sit in my cell watching TV all day. This place is just a waste of my time.'

Brendan looks at Gurman. 'I'll have your telly if you don't like watching it.'

'According to a philosopher called Camus, Sisyphus was a hero,' I say.

Jim looks at me wearily.

I say, 'When Sisyphus was alive, he was a rebel. Death came to cuff him and take him to the underworld, but Sisyphus tricked Death into cuffing his own hands together. Later, when Death finally did claim Sisyphus, Sisyphus managed to sweet-talk the queen of the underworld into letting him go back to the world of the living for an afternoon. He promised he would return to the underworld that night, but he didn't. The gods were offended. They wanted to crush his rebellious spirit. So they made him push the boulder up the hill for eternity.'

'He wasn't a hero for long then, was he?' Jim says.

'Camus thinks Sisyphus can still be a hero even when he's pushing the boulder,' I say.

'How?' Jim says.

'Because Sisyphus doesn't expect that the boulder will stay at the top of the hill, he knows that failure is guaranteed, yet he pushes it to the top anyway. The point at which Sisyphus becomes a hero isn't when he gets to the top—'

'It's when he heads back down,' says Amir.

'Yes. Sisyphus has decided he is going to be happy pushing the rock again. That's his greatest act of rebellion against the gods. He turns the thing that was supposed to make him feel empty and uses it to fill himself up.'

'How can he be happy doing that?' Salvatore says. 'He'd be so angry.'

'Sisyphus isn't angry. Sisyphus is defiant,' Amir says.

'Angry. Defiant. He's still unhappy,' Salvatore says.

Amir squares his shoulders. 'If he's angry, it means he hasn't accepted his situation. You can't be happy if you haven't accepted your situation. Defiance is where you accept your situation, but you carry on anyway. Sisyphus is happy because he's defiant.'

The door opens. Adamson comes in with an A-Board whiteboard. The men stop talking now an officer is in here. He sets up the A-Board, checking to see the legs are even and it won't wobble.

It seems that if I ask Officer Adamson for something, he will emphatically say no, but once I have let him say no and allowed him to go into exacting detail as to why it is he's saying no, he will come back later and give me the thing I asked for, by which time I have come to live without it.

'Thank you,' I say. He leaves without so much as a nod.

Twenty minutes later, Amir is sketching out a picture of Sisyphus pushing the boulder in his notepad. Salvatore rubs his face with his hands like he is scrubbing it. He still hasn't touched his water.

'What happens if Sisyphus says fuck it, I don't want to push this boulder any more?' Jim says.

'The gods would put him on basic,' Brendan says.

'If Sisyphus had a choice between pushing the rock and doing nothing, I bet he'd push the rock,' Gurman says.

'Sisyphus would just be hoping for it to end,' Salvatore says.

I say, 'Camus said that if Sisyphus started hoping for the task to end, then he wouldn't be able to face the demands of his task.'

'Because if Sisyphus is hoping, then there's doubt in his mind,' Amir says. 'Like he's not convinced of his own defiance. If he hopes the boulder will stay at the top, then he'll feel euphoric when he reaches the peak, but he'll feel depressed when he watches it roll back down. It's because he doesn't have hope he can walk down the hill, feeling happy. Because he doesn't hope, he's constantly achieving.'

Salvatore lowers his eyelids. His eyelashes are moist with the beginnings of tears. Amir looks away from him.

I point at the drawing of Sisyphus in the middle of the

circle. 'If Sisyphus told you he was happy, would you believe him?'

Salvatore says, 'I can imagine the boulder rolling down the hill and Sisyphus shouting across to the man on the next mountain pushing a boulder, "Fucking miserable, isn't it? Camus has gone and told everyone I'm happy."'

The men look away from him. Gurman tries not to giggle when he hears the crack of emotion in Salvatore's voice. Jim is palpably pissed off at Salvatore's despair.

I point to the cup of water next to Salvatore's chair.

'Drink, Salvatore. You have to look after yourself now,' I say.

A month later, I'm at my nan's house, having a piss in the bathroom. The toilet is clean white porcelain and smells of lemon bleach.

I finish, go into the living room and sit next to my uncle on the sofa. His belly fills out his T-shirt. He's watching a film called *The Revenant*. It's about a man trying to survive alone in a frozen wilderness. On the screen, Leonardo DiCaprio guts a dead horse and climbs inside it to sleep. Frank's face rests in a gentle smile.

I ask him, 'That borstal you were in, where you were digging those holes – did you ever run out of defiance? Did you ever just hope it would stop?'

He turns from the screen and says, 'The thing was, Andy, you fucking hated it, but that meant you sort of loved it at the same time. It was so full-on that you had to be full-on too. There was no time to wish you was doing something else.'

'What about when you went back to your cell? When

there was no officer there for you to pretend that you loved it to, how did you feel then?'

'I slept like a log. I'd been digging all day.'

'What about when you woke up? You were in a concrete cell.'

'The screws woke me up. I sprang out of bed and said, "Let's do it."'

He looks back at the screen.

Today was a clear day, but now the sky is getting dark. Frank and I didn't make it to the coast. We sit on the sofa, watching telly. He's in his tracksuit bottoms and flip-flops and he drinks tea and smokes roll-ups.

The film is interrupted by an ad break. Frank turns to me again. 'I was only in the seg for a week anyway. After they took me back to the main landing they called out my name at feeding time, but I still wouldn't march, so they covered my plate in salt again. I still wouldn't march though.'

'You really did love digging holes, huh?'

'Then one day I strolled down and they handed me my food and it didn't have any salt on it.'

'You'd earned their respect.'

'They'd given up on me. The geezer handed me my plate and I turned to the screw and said, "You're kidding me! Where's my fucking salt?"'

Time

> I'm teasing you! No better way of passing
> the time when waiting.
> Teasing makes time trip up.
>
> JOHN BERGER

Since I first visited my brother in jail twenty-five years ago, the prison population has doubled, but the amount of space hasn't. Bunk beds have been put into single cells. Cells built to hold two single beds have become triples. The increase in numbers is mostly down to convictions for historical crimes and longer sentences.

A few months ago, a man called Lucus was in my class. He was in his mid-thirties and had light blond hair that he had to keep pushing away from his eyes. He had been offered several appointments at the prison barbers, but never felt like going. He could confidently pronounce the ancient Greek terms we used in class, but he hardly ever accepted my invitation to speak. Most sessions, he sat at a table copying out selected passages from the Bible onto sheets of lined paper. He filled a wad of pages with cramped handwriting. A month or so later, he was doing the same with the Quran.

One week he sat in my class copying out from the Lotus Sutra. I laughed and said, 'That will use up your whole notepad. The Buddhist canon is big enough to fill a small library.' Lucus didn't laugh back. He just kept one finger on the page of the book whilst his other hand kept writing across the paper.

At the end of the class, another student told me that Lucus was serving an IPP sentence. I understood why Lucus didn't laugh back.

People imprisoned for public protection (IPP) have been given a minimum sentence of, say, five years, but the state has the right to hold them on licence for ninety-nine years. After his five years is served, he can apply to a parole board to be released. If the board says no, he has to stay inside and try again two years later. The IPP sentence was introduced in 2005 and was intended for the most serious offences. The government expected to issue 200–300 IPP sentences, but instead there were over 8,000. Some people have been given IPP sentences for shoplifting, stealing a phone or committing criminal damage of less than £20. In 2012 they were abolished, but the abolition was not retrospective. People like Lucus have no idea how long they will be in prison.

In the ancient Greek myth, Zeus wanted to give his father Chronos the most maddening punishment he could contrive, so he made Chronos count all the seconds and minutes and hours, on and on, into eternity. The IPP sentence is Chronos's torture written into law. In 2007, a nineteen-year-old boy called Shane Stroughton was given a two-and-a-half-year tariff and an IPP sentence of ninety-nine years. Ten years later, he was found hanging in his cell.

Lucus kept coming to my class for another couple of months, bringing the Lotus Sutra with him. He never said very much and I didn't press him to talk more. I carried on teaching as normal, occasionally glancing over to make sure he was still copying out passages from transcendental scriptures.

The week after finishing my class on Sisyphus, I'm in a low-security prison, talking to a grey-haired security officer called Davis on the landing. Davis has a good relationship with most men on the landing. I once had a student who was coming up for release who wrote him a two-page letter during my class. It read, 'Thank YOU for seeing the potential in me. Thank YOU for keeping me safe.' He had gone over the word 'YOU' five or six times with his pen.

Davis says, 'Skinner on G-wing was telling me about your class the other day, asking me all of these questions about how do we know if we're free or not. Proper messed me up, it did. I'd love to come and sit in your class for ten minutes. I'd love to hear what they think about the world.'

He tells me about a man called Frederick, who two months ago went to his appeal hearing only to have his sentence lengthened. Since then, he doesn't want to do any class, job or activity the prison has offered him. Davis says, 'I'm a bit worried about him. He's gone quiet. I'd like to sign him up for your class. I don't know how much he'd take part, but honestly, just the walk from his cell to the classroom would be something for him.'

The next week, Frederick comes into my classroom. One of his eyes is half-shut from a fight he had on the landing as a teenager a decade ago. His polo shirt is faded and starched, but he buttons it all the way to the top, as if to guard against whichever indignity will come next. On his right arm, he has lines and lines of tallies tattooed from his elbow upwards, disappearing under the sleeve of his T-shirt. I ask him what they are. He rolls his sleeve to his shoulder. There are forty-six marks. He got them tattooed a few years ago when he had just been released from serving forty-six months.

I get the class underway. I tell the men about the paradox of Zeno's arrow. 'Zeno says that before the arrow can reach its target, it will have to first travel half of the distance to the target. Then, to travel the remaining distance, the arrow will have to first travel half of that remaining distance. Once it has done that, it will have to travel the remaining distance by first travelling half of it.'

The men groan.

'Even when it gets to one millimetre away from the target, it will have to travel half a millimetre before it reaches the target. Then it will have to travel half of half a millimetre. And half of what's left, and half of what's left again after that. Zeno says that the arrow will never hit the target. However close it gets, it will always have half of the remaining distance left to travel.'

The men discuss the paradox. Most of them find it annoying. They keep saying: 'It will hit the target, though.' 'In real life it will.' 'It will just get really close and then it will get closer and hit the target. It's going to hit the target.'

The men look irritated and disengaged, so I call a fifteen-minute break. They go out into the corridor to vape. I go and stand with them. I notice more tallies poking out from the bottom of the T-shirt sleeve of Frederick's left arm too. He catches me looking and rolls up his sleeve to show me. There are only about two dozen tallies.

'When I came here this time, I started marking this sentence,' he says. 'Each month, I'd add a line. But I'd feel so depressed afterwards when I saw how much blank skin there was left on my arm. So I started adding a line at the end of each week. That made me feel even worse. I gave up in the end.'

My friend David Breakspear has done several years inside. When he was a teenager, he and his mates would call the police to report themselves, put the phone down and run. By the time he was in his twenties, prison was like a home to him. Recently, he told me, 'People would say to me "Don't do the crime, if you can't do the time." But I wanted to do the time. The crime was a means to an end. Punishment was the reward.' I asked him how he used to pass the hours in jail. 'Having a night out,' he said. 'A night out' is a euphemism for getting high. At five o'clock, the guards would lock him up for the night, he'd smoke some heroin and be taken into a reality where time didn't exist. When he came to, he started glugging water. He knew that if he got asked to do a piss test and they found heroin in his system then the prison would keep him inside for an extra thirty days. Going for a night out was a gamble; it could kill time but it might also add more of it to his sentence. Heroin typically shows up in a piss test for seventy-two hours after use, but David necked enough water to make sure he was pissing every twenty minutes – his proven method for flushing the drugs out of his system by twelve o'clock the next day.

David was last released from prison shortly before turning fifty and has spent the last five years passionately working as a prison reform campaigner. Today, his daily routine is the same as how it used to be when he was inside. At home, he wakes up, goes to sleep, eats his food and has a nap in time with the regime. 'But I no longer need a night out,' he said. 'I got so many projects on the go, I wish there were more hours in the day.'

At the weekend, I'm home sat at my desk, looking on my laptop for ideas for classes. I come across an article that says in the sixties, Samuel Beckett's play *Waiting for Godot* was performed at San Quentin prison in California. It was staged in a boxing ring positioned where the trapdoors of the gallows once were.

In my early twenties, I booked tickets for two different Samuel Beckett plays – *Krapp's Last Tape* and *Not I* – a month apart from each other. Excited to be experiencing the monumental Beckett for the first time, I went to the theatre and took my seat for *Krapp's Last Tape*. The lights went down and I watched an old man in a dingy room listen to recordings of himself and then make more recordings of himself. The play finished. Relieved, I left the theatre and went to the Italian place a few doors down and ate a tiramisu. A month later, on the day I was due to go and see *Not I*, I came home from work and put the TV on. I'd heard that *Not I* was set on a pitch-black stage where only the actress's mouth was illuminated. The mouth spoke at a ferocious pace in jumbled sentences. A couple of hours later, when I should have been setting off to the theatre, a *Friends* marathon started on the telly. I picked up my phone and asked the pizza place to deliver me a margherita.

At my laptop, I scroll down and keep reading the article. The author talks about Rick Cluchey, a man who discovered Beckett whilst doing time in San Quentin. Upon release, Cluchey became friends with the playwright and performed in *Waiting for Godot* under Beckett's direction. Beckett scholar Lance Duerfahrd claimed Cluchey 'was able to inhabit a Beckett character in ways people who'd been through acting school can only dream to attain'.

I look up from my laptop and gaze into the middle distance. Now is normally the time they show old episodes of *The Simpsons* on one of the Freeview channels.

I look back at the screen and try to focus. I download a copy of *Waiting for Godot* and make some notes.

Two days later, I'm in my classroom. A man called Ziggy is the first person to arrive. He has a narrow face and a wide moustache that turns up at the ends. Today, he's carrying an extra T-shirt in his hand. He slouches into a chair and then places the T-shirt over his face.

'Are you OK, Ziggy?' I say.

He half lifts up the T-shirt on his head, as if it is a veil, and says, 'Did we have this lesson yesterday?'

'Yesterday was Sunday,' I say.

'A ghost was talking with me all night. I've hardly slept.'

'He doesn't sound very considerate.'

Ziggy's elbows are pointing up and out as he holds the T-shirt. 'Actually, they were delightful.'

'Was it a female ghost?' I ask.

''This is a men's prison,' Ziggy says.

'Was he in ghost prison?'

Ziggy tuts. 'My cell is right by where the gallows used to be.'

'Always good to meet the neighbours,' I say.

'He was a decent bloke, I could tell.'

'I wonder why they hanged him.'

'I didn't like to ask.' Ziggy lowers the T-shirt back over his face and folds his arms.

A moment later, Wayne comes in. Wayne is doing an indefinite sentence. He was given a six-year tariff thirteen years ago. In the prison where he was before transferring to this one four months ago, he attended the fashion class so he could get out of his cell. Each lesson, he worked on a pair of trousers he was making, but twenty minutes before the end of each class, he unstitched some of the work he'd done so that he could keep attending. Wayne's transfer came suddenly before he had finished the trousers. The fashion teacher in his last prison put it in an envelope and sent it here. Wayne received it last week.

Wayne doesn't sit down but stands behind his chair instead. He asks me, 'How old are you?'

'Thirty-two,' I say.

'How the fuck can you be thirty-two? I'm thirty-eight!'

Wayne looks at Ziggy sitting with a T-shirt over his head and looks back at me.

'Chatty cellmate,' I say.

'I'm sharing with a dickhead,' Wayne says. 'He only got himself nicked because he's homeless and he wants a bed for the winter. Last night he started moaning because he got a letter saying he was being let out in December for good behaviour. He knows I'm an IPP, but he kept whinging about how he doesn't want to leave.'

Ziggy lifts the shirt off his face. 'You don't want to be IPP. I gave up violent crime after IPP came in. That's a horrible sentence.'

'I am a fucking IPP,' Wayne says.

'Oh, wow.' Ziggy lowers the T-shirt back over his face.

A moment later, Wim arrives. He's a Dutch man in his early forties who has been successfully detoxing from drugs for the last nine months. He has long flowing hair and looks ten years younger than he does in the mugshot on his prison-issued ID card. He does a double take at seeing Ziggy. 'Are we in Abu Ghraib?'

'Someone kept him up all night,' I say.

'Last week, they put a nineteen-year-old in with me for just one night,' Wim says. 'He was getting bailed in the morning, but he couldn't handle it. He was up the whole night, every ten minutes he was pressing the buzzer asking the guvs, "You know I'm going to court tomorrow, right?" And then again twenty minutes later, buzzing it: "Are you sure I'm on the paperwork to go to court tomorrow? Don't forget, yeah!" He finally fell asleep. I was too pissed off to sleep. I kept imagining myself shouting at him, telling him not to waste his life.'

Wim walks over to Ziggy's chair and says, 'Who are you sharing with, Ziggy?'

'I'm a single cell.' Ziggy's words are muffled by the T-shirt.

Wim scratches his head. He moves his lips as if about to say something but just sits down instead.

The last few men come in and take their seats in the circle. Andrew is the last person to come in, a British-Jamaican man in his early thirties. He wears glasses that are fixed up with Sellotape on both arms. It's been fourteen days since I've spoken to him. In these fourteen days, he has been released and returned to prison. I hadn't noticed that he'd left.

'I'm so angry with myself for being back here,' he says.

'I'm sorry. How long till you get out again?' I ask.

'Ten months.' He sighs. 'I'm hoping it will go quickly, though. That's the strange thing about coming to prison. From the second you get sentenced, you realize how precious time is, and so you start wishing time away because you want to get out again.'

Andrew takes a seat. I close the door.

'The playwright Samuel Beckett lived in Paris, opposite a prison,' I say. 'He could see over the wall from his window. He would stand on his balcony and communicate to men in their cells using a light and a mirror.'

'Was he a drug dealer?' Wim says.

'He wrote a play where two old men called Didi and Gogo, wearing bedraggled suits, are standing next to a dead tree. They're waiting for a man called Godot to arrive. They wait all day. Just before sundown, a child comes and tells them Mr Godot won't come today but he will come tomorrow. The sun goes down and Didi and Gogo keep waiting.'

Ziggy adjusts the T-shirt on his head to make sure it doesn't fall off.

'Didi and Gogo wait for the whole of the next day. Just before nightfall, the child comes back again and tells them that Mr Godot won't be coming today, but he will surely come tomorrow. Didi tells the child that's what he said yesterday, but the boy claims he didn't come yesterday, that it must have been his brother who came instead. The boy leaves. Gogo says, "I can't go on like this." "That's what you think," Didi replies.'

Wayne narrows his eyes at me.

I say, 'Time drags. Didi and Gogo are desperate for distraction. Throughout the play, they plead to each other: "What do we do now?", "What'll we do?" and "What should we do whilst we wait?"'

'What do they do?' asks Andrew.

'They try lots of things. At one point, they try to pass the time by fighting each other,' I say.

'The two in the cell next to me were proper fighting last night,' Wim says. 'The guards had to separate them. One wanted to watch BBC and the other wanted to watch ITV.'

Andrew says, 'You know when you first come to prison, you get a TV in your cell and you think "I'm saved". But now it's just all repeats.'

Andrew starts talking about a row between two characters on last night's episode of *EastEnders*. Wim joins in. Pockets of the class talk about *The Simpsons* and *Love Island*. I put my hand up to get the class's attention. They notice, but almost all of them are now talking about telly. I lower my hand and lean back in my chair, waiting for them to finish. They talk about *Hollyoaks*, *Family Guy* and a documentary series called *Inside the World's Toughest Prisons*.

I lean back in my chair for three or four minutes, waiting for the telly conversation to fizzle out. When it does, I sit up and continue with the lesson about *Waiting for Godot*. 'Didi and Gogo try to kill time by sleeping. But they hate it when the other one starts dreaming.'

'Sleep is the longest way to do your sentence. It's like doing prison underwater,' Wim says.

Ziggy half lifts up his T-shirt. 'I didn't get any sleep last night.'

'Why don't Didi and Gogo just leave?' Wayne says.

'At one point, they agree to leave, but then they just keep standing there,' I say.

'What even is Godot?' Wayne says.

'Didi and Gogo aren't sure what Godot looks like. They try to remember why Godot wanted to meet them, but they can't remember. They can just about recall that Godot said he could only offer "nothing very definite" and that he "couldn't promise anything".'

'So it's just a trick then. Godot isn't anything.'

'We are all waiting,' Wim says. 'Maybe for God or to die. For an epiphany.'

'You think this is something deep, Wim, but I swear it's not,' Wayne says. 'Godot is like the monster in a horror movie. You're always afraid of it because you never see it, you just sense it. Horror filmmakers are clever like that, but it's nothing deep. Beckett is just trying to play with you.'

'Maybe we don't even know what you're waiting for, you're just waiting for that thing that will make sense of the reason we've been waiting,' Wim says.

'That sounds deep, but I don't have a clue what you're talking about,' Wayne says.

Wim runs his hands through his hair. 'When I was begging, the worst thing I could do was lose patience. If you lose your temper or sound sarcastic, then nobody gives you money. It don't matter how many rejections you get, you gotta just keep on.'

Wayne scoffs and shakes his head.

I say, 'Didi tries telling a joke to pass the time. But just before he gets to the punchline, he has to go off to piss because he has a weak prostate. Later, Didi tries to sing a song about the death of a dog but keeps forgetting the lyrics. Everything they try either fails, backfires or quickly runs out of steam.'

'They could remind themselves that they could kill themselves if they need to,' Wayne says. 'I'm not saying they should kill themselves. But just knowing it's an option makes things easier.'

I say, 'At the end of the play, they pull at either end of Gogo's belt to test if it's strong enough to hang themselves with. It snaps and the two almost fall over. Gogo's trousers fall to his ankles and the play ends.'

Wayne flares his nostrils. 'Beckett is just trying to fuck with us.'

I ask the class, 'How should Didi and Gogo wait for Godot?'

'Maybe Godot is still coming; he's just on BPT – black people time,' Andrew says.

Some of the other black students laugh.

Andrew's glasses wobble as he talks. 'If a black person says he's gonna meet you at twelve, that means he'll set off at about half one and he'll still be an hour early. That's my theory about why they can put so many of us in jail and we don't rise up. We don't care about time. Honestly, Didi and Gogo should try waiting for Godot in Jamaica.'

Ziggy is still slouched in his chair with a T-shirt over his head. Wayne looks increasingly irritated.

Wim moves his hair out the way of his eyes and says, 'If Didi and Gogo are always looking down the road to see if Godot is coming, then they'll go mad. But they'll also go mad if they try not to think about Godot any more. That's like trying not to think of pink elephants. So they shouldn't think about him and they shouldn't avoid thinking about him.'

'How can they do that?' Wayne says.

'Distract themselves.'

'That's the same as avoiding thinking about him,' Wayne says, his bottom teeth edging forward.

'Avoiding thinking about Godot means Godot is always at the centre of their minds. Distracting themselves means they've forgotten about him for a bit. It's like me in here. I'll write out an app for a job, and weeks later, I'm asking every officer I see to chase it up. I want my response yesterday, but I always have to wait until tomorrow to get the answer I don't want. I can drive myself mad unless I distract myself from thinking about my app.'

'Didi and Gogo have nothing to distract themselves with,' Wayne says.

'They could always get the kid to bring them an ounce when he comes back tomorrow,' Wim says.

Everyone in the room laughs.

'I'd beat the shit out of Didi and Gogo,' Wayne says.

'Yes, Didi and Gogo are the problem,' Wim says. 'If I was there waiting, I'd stay away from them and keep myself to myself. Their panic and complaining would just bring me down. You just need to stay in your own head where you can take control of time, not like those two. Time has taken control of them.'

'How can Didi and Gogo take control of time?' I ask.

Wim says, 'When Didi and Gogo wake up, they should try to make it till noon. At noon they should try and make it to early evening, then try and make it to night-time. If that doesn't work, then just try and make it through the next hour or the next twenty minutes. Or the next two minutes.'

Wayne screws up his face. 'Then the kid comes and tells them they have to do it all over again. The thing I hate most about prison is when I ask a screw for something and they tell me to ask them again tomorrow. Then the next day I ask and they aren't here. They're on holiday or it's not their shift. I wish they wouldn't fucking lie to me. Just tell me no. I can live with no.'

I ask Wayne, 'What do you think Didi and Gogo should say to the kid?'

'Ignore him,' Wayne says.

Wim stretches his arms. Andrew asks the man next to him for the time. The energy in the room is fizzling out. Ziggy takes the T-shirt off his head, yawns and says, 'Are we still talking about those two beggars?'

'We're discussing how Didi and Gogo should wait,' Wim says.

'Depends when the bloke is getting there,' Ziggy says.

'They don't know,' Wayne says.

'They must know. Otherwise, why would they still be there?' Ziggy says.

'They don't know when he's coming,' Wayne says.

'Well, they need to find out when he will come.'

'Big man, you weren't listening. They can't fucking know. That's the whole point of the stupid story.'

'I was asleep for that bit.'

'Then why are you even offering your opinion?' Wayne says.

'They should definitely find out when he's coming,' Ziggy

says. 'Uncertainty isn't good. If he's not coming, they should just leave.'

'Why don't you go back to sleep,' Wayne says. He stands up and walks out of the room, slamming the door behind him.

We all look at each other. Wim pulls an awkward face.

'They should just follow the kid. That'll lead them to Godot,' Ziggy says.

I tell the men to talk amongst themselves for a moment. I go and look through the glass of the door. Wayne is pacing up and down in the corridor. He's muttering under his breath. Behind me, Andrew and Wim talk about *Love Island*. Someone mentions *Dragons' Den*. The volume in the room goes up. Everyone talks about telly.

Madness

> For you must know, my dear ones, that each of
> us is undoubtedly guilty on behalf of all and
> for all on earth.
>
> DOSTOYEVSKY

Over the last two months I've been afraid I will burn my house down. Most mornings I step out of the front door, walk to the end of my street and think I have left the stove on. I tell myself that I have not left the stove on, but I think, what if I return home after work to find the fire brigade putting out the fire raging through the building? My housemates' charred bodies are being zipped up into bags and taken away.

I run back home to check I have turned the oven off. Sometimes I have to run back home a second time to check that I checked properly the first time. Even if I have not used the stove that morning, the executioner in my head tells me I must have done something bad. The dread is too intense, I have to go back and make sure that I haven't.

To save time, I have taken to photographing the stove before I leave the house. Now when I walk to the end of the street and panic that I have left the stove on, I can look at my phone and confirm that I haven't. Sometimes looking at the photo puts me at ease and my executioner thoughts quiet down. But on other days that doesn't make the dread go away. It's as though the guilt is so fundamental that it doesn't need any content. It's nebulous, like a toxic gas smothering me.

Three months ago, on a beautiful summer day, I took a canal boat out down the river with Johnny, my friend of twenty years. Whenever we saw a weeping willow leaning out across the water, we piloted the boat through its dangling branches. We giggled every time the leaves brushed over our heads. Last night, I took out my phone to look at photos of that day. I had to scroll up on my camera past almost sixty images of my oven before I got to the river.

Today, I am waiting in my classroom to teach a group of Vulnerable Prisoners (VPs) – people who might get their heads smashed in should they mix with the other prisoners. Many VPs are in for sexual offences, but some are put on the wing because they have drug debts or are at risk from gangs in the mainstream prison population. This classroom has big windows that look out onto the landing. The glass is reinforced. Security tell me that I have to keep the door locked at all times. If certain mainstream prisoners got inside the room, then it would be a 'bloodbath'. However, I must always keep the window blinds open, so the guards can keep an eye on the class in case VPs attack each other.

A group of seven VPs arrive, escorted by two guards. The students come in and sit in two groups at the opposite ends of the room. The group on the left side of the room are thirty years younger than the group on the right. Most debtors on the VP wing are teenagers or in their early twenties. A lot of the rest of the men are in their fifties and sixties.

The officers leave and lock the door behind them.

Ash and Devon sit next to each other. Ash was a geography professor before he was inside. He's thirty years older than me and twice as educated. He wears a red-and-blue checked long-sleeve shirt that I can easily picture him wearing in a classroom. Once, during June, I took some reading to his cell and I saw that he still had a Christmas card next to his bed.

Devon wears a pair of prison issue shoes and a T-shirt with an image of a palm tree and sunset on the front. He's nearly forty but cannot read. I think he has undiagnosed learning disability. Last week some of the men were talking about Saturn. Devon looked confused. He thought that Saturn was the same thing as the moon. When they told him Saturn and the moon were different things he got angry with them because he thought they were trying to tease him. Today, Devon has brought a legal letter to the class and Ash is explaining it to him. Ash tries to teach him how to pronounce a word. Devon says, 'Ssss . . .' He squints at the page. 'Sss-u-lisss-itt-or.'

From the other side of the room, someone says 'Nonces' as they fake cough. The young men sat next to him laugh. Edo is nineteen and has told everyone he's in for drug crime and was only transferred to the VP wing because of beefs on the wing, but in fact he's in for a sexual offence.

Half a dozen men being transported back to their cells pass outside the window. One bangs the glass and shouts 'Fucking nonces'. Edo bends forward in his chair, unties his shoelaces and ties them back up again, hiding his face in the process. He checks for the men to pass before he sits back up again.

*

The men are looking at me, waiting for the lesson to start. With mainstream prisoners, it takes ages to get them to stop chatting and pay attention, but these men don't like talking to each other.

I say, 'There's a story in the Bible where Jesus goes to the temple and finds moneylenders are working there. He makes a whip of cords and drives them out. He throws their tables over and tells them to "not make my Father's house a house of trade".'

'I believe the line is, "Do not make my Father's house into a den of robbers,"' Ash says.

'Apologies, Ash. A den of robbers,' I say.

'Why did Jesus throw the tables over?' Devon says.

'Because he's angry,' Ash says.

'Why?' Devon says.

'Because they're doing business in the temple and a temple is a sacred place,' Ash says.

'What's sacred mean?'

'Sacred is when something is special and it should never be damaged.'

'Urgh!' Alfie says, his lip curling in disgust. Alfie is on the VP wing because of a drug debt. He's about nineteen.

I try to get a conversation going about the cleansing of the temple, but the men keep sniping at each other. A few minutes into the class, I already feel drained.

One man in the class, Louis, has an uncannily similar-looking face to my first girlfriend's dad. He was a second-hand car salesman who wore gold rings on both hands and had a sunbed tan. Each time I see Louis, I'm momentarily struck by how sallow he is in comparison. Louis doesn't like Ash and hasn't since our first class together when Ash said, 'I learnt how to survive prison by going to boarding school,' and Louis retorted, 'I learnt how to survive prison by growing up on a council estate.'

I try to keep the class going. 'Jesus drove the lenders from the temple. What other places should the market stay out of? In California, men in prison can pay $82 to spend the night in a luxury cell. On the internet, you can pay a professional apologizer to write a "sorry" letter on your behalf.'

'Money can make any problem go away,' Louis says.

Ash shakes his head.

Louis says, 'There are people who've done exactly what I'm in for, but they haven't gone to prison because they can just pay their way out of it, out of court.'

'That doesn't make the problem go away,' Ash says.

Louis leans forward in his chair and says, 'Rich people live longer. They eat well.'

'That's nothing to do with money. McDonald's is far more expensive than fresh fruit and vegetables,' Ash says.

'You don't understand poverty.'

'People need to learn how to control themselves.'

Louis gets out of his chair and closes the blinds. I walk over to the window to open them again.

'We're allowed to close them,' Louis says.

'The officer said we have to keep them open,' I say.

'Half the screws are corrupt anyway,' Louis says.

I open the blinds.

Over the next half-hour, I keep throwing new ideas into the conversation to keep the pace moving so there is less opportunity for bickering. I say, 'There's a controversial charity in the US. It pays women who are addicted to heroin $300 to be sterilized.'

'Doesn't that bring up questions of consent?' Ash says.

Edo nudges Alfie. The two laugh.

'What are you laughing at?' Devon says.

'They're laughing at nothing, Devon. Don't listen to them,' Ash says.

A week later, I take a photo of my stove, leave the house and travel to prison. On my walk to work, I feel a sense of doom. I take out my phone and look at today's photo of the oven, but it doesn't reassure me. The executioner tells me that even if I haven't done something wrong, then I will soon. There's nothing I can do to change it. It's too late to fight. The best thing I can do is go quietly.

An hour later, in my classroom, I open the blinds. There are three rows of tables across the room. I drop my rucksack on the floor, push the tables against the wall and make a circle of chairs in the middle of the class. An officer comes in and tells me there has been a change of location for philosophy. The tables have been set up in rows because the room is going to be used as a call centre to give the men work experience. Men will make computer-generated calls and ask people to participate in market research questionnaires. They'll be paid around £3 a day to do it.

I pick up my bag and step towards the door.

'Before you go,' the officer says, 'please put the tables back.'

I put the tables back, lock the room and walk through the prison towards my new location. On the wall in the corridor is a display with forty or fifty different portrait photos on it. They're the faces of ex-prisoners that the prison invites each month to talk to the men about life after crime. People who used to be inside for drug dealing, armed robbery, gang crime or murder tell how they became marathon runners, prize-winning artists, business entrepreneurs, youth centre workers, university lecturers or published authors. They come in as inspirational examples to men that they too can turn their vices into virtues. None of the portraits are of sex offenders.

I come to a security gate and go into the office to sign in. An officer in his late fifties is leaning back in his chair, holding a cup of tea. He's a terse Yorkshireman called Stiles. Another officer about my age is doing some paperwork at a desk. I open the signing-in book.

'Are you healthcare?' Stiles says.

'I'm doing philosophy with VPs,' I say.

'Philosophy? With those people? Those people are animals,' he says.

I grimace. I imagine how it must feel to live in a cell when the man who has the key to your door thinks you're an animal. I imagine myself locked in such a cell. The executioner tells me that's where I should be.

The younger officer speaks up. 'What are we supposed to do, just give them bread and water?'

'Would you let them babysit your children, would you?' Stiles says.

'That doesn't matter. We still have to look after them,' the younger one says.

I write my name and details in the logbook and leave the officers to their argument.

I go to my classroom. I open the blinds and wait for my

class to arrive. Fifteen minutes later, crowds of men are walking past the window. They're mainstream prisoners. I'll have to wait until they have been transported to their location and locked inside before the officers unlock the VPs and bring them over. The two groups aren't allowed to move through the landing at the same time. For the same reason, VPs have to travel back to their cells earlier than other men.

I clean my whiteboard. My whiteboard pens are lined up on my desk in the order of red, black, green and blue. I reorder them to black, blue, red and green. I wait.

When I was a teenager, I knew somewhere inside me that the executioner in my head was irrational and I tried to tell myself that I'd done nothing wrong. But around that time, the *News of the World* printed the names, photographs and believed whereabouts of convicted paedophiles. Shortly after, 150 people rioted outside the flat of one man named in the newspaper. They threw stones at his window, overturned a car and set it on fire. They threw a brick into a policeman's face. Elsewhere in England, other people named in the paper were attacked. Some were paedophiles, others merely shared the same name as a paedophile. I felt queasy when I switched on the television and saw that vigilantes had graffitied the word 'paedo' across the house of a paediatrician. It didn't matter if I knew the executioner in my head was irrational; the TV was showing me I could be punished for no reason.

I've been waiting forty minutes for the VPs to arrive. Bored of sitting in my chair, I meander up and down my empty classroom. There's a copy of the *Inside Time* on my desk, a newspaper for people inside. I sit at the desk and open it. On one page, there are numerous adverts for law firms specializing in appeals. On the next page, there's an advert stating that if you've had an accident in prison in the last two years that wasn't your fault, then you could be entitled to several thousand pounds.

I find an article about a middle-aged man who recently died of cirrhosis of the liver. He had been in a youth detention centre in the eighties, where he was raped by one of the officers, a man called Neville Husband. Husband was believed to have sexually assaulted over 300 boys whilst he worked in prisons. He targeted children that had grown up in care and had no family support. One victim says Husband apologized after each time he raped him, promising not to do it again and then threatening the boy that they'd be found dead in a cell if they told anyone. Numerous officers knew what Husband was doing but did nothing.

I close the paper. I feel nauseous and I feel a strange sense of shame. Working in prison, I can't forget that I'm working for an institution that often dehumanizes and traumatizes people to a degree that is as harmful as the offences they were sentenced for. When I read about abuses of power, I almost feel complicit.

The door opens. It's Officer Stiles, with a line of VPs behind him. He ushers them into the room. I close the paper.

'Radio me if any of them give you trouble. I'll take care of it,' Stiles says to me.

I don't say anything back, a failed attempt to avoid complicity.

Stiles shuts the door, locks it and walks off. The men take their seats. There are only five men this week. Alfie has been kicked off the VP wing for bullying a paedophile. He was sent back to the main part of the prison, but he still has debts to drug dealers there, so he has been put in a cell with an officer positioned outside full-time to guard him.

Louis walks over to the window and closes the blinds. I walk over to open them again, but Louis accosts me.

He says, 'Andy, I wanted to say, I think there's something about you that's very special. The way you tell stories, the way you hold yourself. I was trying to think of which actor you reminded me of the other day. I couldn't decide if you looked more like Christian Bale or Tom Cruise. You've got a gift. I see more than just teaching in your future. I think you could be an actor.'

'I like teaching, Louis,' I say.

'I know you do, and that's great. But I just get upset that more of the world cannot see your talent. Why don't you let me introduce you to some of my associates?'

'I can't do that, Louis,' I say.

'I'm talking TV, film, musicals, Andy. I know people who could make you famous. I don't say this to everyone I meet, but I see big things for you.'

'Thank you, Louis, but that can't happen,' I say.

'Don't feel as though you have to answer today. Think about it for a bit.'

I open the blinds.

I get the lesson underway, but I feel lethargic. When I teach mainstream prisoners, I enjoy the buzz of being in a group of men talking together. I don't experience such fraternal feeling with VPs. I'm more formal. It's partly because I want to keep my distance so Louis can't cross my boundaries, but maybe, like Stiles, I'm conceited enough to believe I'm a different species to these men.

Edo doesn't call anyone a 'nonce' this week. He's quiet. I ask him questions, but he gives one-word answers. I ask him to say more, but he giggles nervously. The less he says, the less likely he is to get found out. He's helped by the fact that there's a culture of silence amongst these VPs. Many mainstream prisoners will talk casually about how they are in for fraud, or they'll proudly call themselves a drug dealer, but VPs hardly ever talk about their crimes. On the rare occasion they do, it's either with denial, minimization and self-victimization, or with intense shame. I try to take the conversation back to philosophy.

Thirty minutes into the lesson, Ash comes in. He has been in a meeting with his resettlement officer, talking about what job he could do after release. When he first started having these meetings last month, he was still hoping he would be able to work in education by marking exams online. However, he wasn't sure if the terms of his release allowed him to have an internet connection. After another meeting, he said he'd be happy working on a building site, but another man laughed and said, 'Till someone googles you.' 'I wish the internet had never been invented,' someone said. This week, Ash tells the man sitting next to him that he's going to apply for a job in an animal rescue centre.

A few minutes later, I say to the class, 'Derrida thought that only unforgivable acts were worthy of forgiveness.'

'That doesn't make sense to me,' Ash says.

'He says to forgive, we have to forget ordinary logic. He says what makes forgiveness special is that it's not weighed or calculated. It's one of life's only genuine surprises.'

'How are you supposed to do that?' Ash says.

'Derrida says you need to access a kind of madness to forgive.'

'Was he a psycho? I know blokes like that on the wing. They do something evil one minute and forget about it the next.'

'Do you think forgiveness requires a kind of madness?' I ask.

'I spend every minute I'm in this place trying not to go mad.'

I tell the men a story. 'Simon Wiesenthal was a Jewish architect incarcerated in Lemberg Concentration Camp in 1943. He was taken from the camp to the hospital and to the bedside of a dying Nazi soldier called Karl Seidl. Karl explained how he'd helped cram about 300 Jews into a house and then thrown in grenades. A family tried to escape by jumping out of second-floor windows, but Karl shot them before they could make it out. A few weeks later, Karl was in combat facing Russian artillery fire. He froze in the middle of the battlefield.'

'Oh shit,' Louis says.

'He told Wiesenthal that he "saw the burning family, the father with the child and behind them the mother – and they came to meet me. No, I cannot shoot at them a second time." A shell exploded and Karl lost consciousness.'

Devon is snoring. Ash nudges him and he wakes up.

I say, 'Karl woke up on a hospital ward, soon to die from his injuries. He'd asked for a Jew to be brought to his bedside so he could ask for his forgiveness.'

'Forgiveness for what?' Louis says.

I continue. 'Simon didn't know what to say. He sat with Karl in silence. Karl's breathing got fainter until it stopped and he died. For decades after, Simon was preoccupied with asking philosophers, writers and religious ministers if he should have said something to Seidl.'

Louis throws his hands up in the air and says, 'Karl didn't need to ask for forgiveness.'

'It was abusive of Karl to ask Simon that. He wasn't seeing him as a person but as a Jew,' Ash says.

'If Simon had been born as Karl, he'd have done exactly the same thing,' Louis says.

Ten minutes later, Ash says, 'I don't think it was just that Karl was afraid of dying. I think he truly wanted forgiveness because he knew he'd done something wrong.'

'Why do you think that?' I ask.

Ash explains. 'When he saw the woman and child in the sights of his rifle, he realized what he'd done. He stood frozen because he thought he deserved to die and he wanted a bullet to hit him in the head. That was his plea for forgiveness. But it wasn't enough. That's why he has to wake up and keep going through it.'

'Does that mean he wasn't forgivable?' I ask.

Ash looks past my shoulder.

I turn around. Three men are staring through the window, their foreheads pressed against the glass.

Twenty minutes before free flow, Officer Stiles comes inside my room to collect the men.

'We're in the middle of a conversation,' Ash says to the officer.

'You need to calm down,' the officer says.

Ash clenches his jaw.

The men stand up and file out. Ash shakes my hand and asks me if I could extend the course for another two sessions because of how our classes are shorter than they are for mainstream prisoners. I tell him I need to think about it.

The men leave. I lock the door behind them and fall into my chair. I close my eyes and wait for my blood pressure to come back down.

I'm startled by a bang on the window. I open my eyes and see a man. His bulky fist is pressed against the glass.

He stares at me.

I stare back at him, trying not to show any fear. I'm clenching my thighs.

He narrows his eyes at me, laughs and walks off.

I let out a long sigh. I stretch my legs out to try and relax, but a block of tension remains in my chest.

I think I'm going to say yes to Ash about extending the course, despite the fact I find working in this section of the prison so triggering of the executioner in my head. In fact, it's because I find it so triggering that I want to keep going. I don't want to let the executioner win. I've already let him take too much from me. When I see myself in photos lately, I seem shorter than I used to be, as though I have lost two inches from cowering. I want to stand up tall again. I'm going to carry on with this class and when the toxic gas envelops me, I will prove I can stay on my feet. When the executioner comes, I will stare him out.

A couple of days later, I travel to a rural prison, 200 miles from home. I step off the bus and walk, listening to the mix Spotify has made for me. The opening bars of Michael Jackson's 'Billie Jean' play on my earphones. I can press a little heart on my phone and Spotify will play me more music by Jackson. Alternatively, I can swipe and the app will exclude Jackson from my future mixes.

I come to the gates of the prison. I take out my earphones and switch off the phone.

This prison holds only sex offenders. Inside, there are gardening and bakery courses. I hear classical music coming from some of the cells. The books borrowed in the library are often of a literary flavour, but there are hardly any art history books on account of all the images of infant cherubs. I'm less guarded about my physical space here. There's less violence, self-harm and drugs than in an ordinary prison. Some prison regimes ask staff to refer to the men as 'residents', which I find too Orwellian to comply with, but the number of people wearing linen trousers in this institution makes the word seem fitting.

Thirty minutes later, I'm teaching a class of twenty in the library. The group is really vocal and open with each other. I tell the men about how Prometheus was punished for giving humans fire. For once, I don't have to double-check whether there are any convicted arsonists in the room before I continue with the story.

The class is great fun. At any one time, about ten or twelve men have their hand in the air to speak. The group is cheerful and relaxed. There's an atmosphere of good humour that I don't see with VPs in ordinary prisons. If I want to stare out the executioner, it won't be easy to find him here.

The conversation is still buzzing when the officer tells us it's time for the men to go back to their cells. Several men come up to me and give me a handmade thank you card on behalf of the group.

The men leave. I show the librarian the card.

'The lesson meant a lot to them,' the librarian says.

'Half of them have PhDs. I don't think I taught them much they didn't already know,' I say.

'They loved it. They crave a moment where they can lose themselves.'

The next day, I'm in a mainstream wing of a high-security prison. On the landing, I hear shouting coming from behind me.

'Fuck you! Fuck you!'

I turn around. About five metres behind me, four officers are restraining a man. They lower him to the ground. They put his hands behind his back and cuff him. It's distressing to watch.

'Fuck you!' the man shouts, but quieter this time.

Two more officers run onto the scene. They lift the man to his feet. His face is bright red. He's breathing heavily.

The officers escort him towards the segregation unit. I'm also heading in that direction. I walk behind, following them through a long and otherwise empty corridor. The walls are made of breeze blocks that have been slathered in white emulsion. The man is walking bent over and with his face down. I can't see his head.

I feel queasy. The officers deliberately walk slowly to help de-escalate the tension. I'm forced to walk at a fraction of my normal pace. I think about overtaking the man, but I want to prove I can endure this sight. I stay in his trail.

That night, I'm asleep in bed. I wake with a falling sensation, like my foot is slipping off a kerb. I'm in a foetal position and

I'm hyperventilating. My fingers are curled. I can't straighten them. I try to get out of bed, but it is as if my legs have petrified.

I think about the knives in the kitchen. The executioner tells me I'm going to hurt someone with them. He says that maybe I already have and I've blocked out the memory. I vigilantly go over every day of the last week to make sure I didn't cut anyone. I know my thoughts are absurd, but I'm also confident of my guilt. Even if I didn't harm someone in the past, I cannot be sure I won't do in the future.

The fear peaks and then subsides. My breathing slows and I can move my fingers again. I sit up in bed. I tell myself that I am OK, I have done nothing wrong. I have no desire to hurt anyone. But the executioner is too strong. The fear has such authority. I must in some way be illegal.

My breathing quickens. My fingers curl towards the heel of my hand. My body is crushed with dread once again.

The following morning, I get ready to go to work. I walk into the kitchen and take a photo of the stove. I see a six-inch kitchen knife on the draining rack. I open a drawer, put the knife in the very back and slam the drawer shut.

'For fuck's sake,' I say.

I close my eyes and sigh. This morning, the executioner has won.

A few hours later, I open the blinds in my classroom. The men come in and sit down, but Louis approaches me in the corner of the room and says, 'Andy, I had a new idea for our project: voice-overs. We should get you doing car adverts. You've got a wonderful voice, you know.'

'We should start the lesson,' I say.

'I know some casting directors who would snap you up,' he says.

'I've thought about this, Louis.'

'Fantastic!'

'It can't happen.'

'My associates are some of the top people in that area of business.'

'Can we move on?' I ask.

He makes a face like a grumpy child.

'I think we should have the blinds half open today,' he says.

'They have to be fully open,' I say.

Louis sits down and sulks.

A moment later, I hand Ash, Louis and the others an image of Edward Colston's statue. On the plaque underneath the figure, it says, 'Here stands one of the city's most virtuous men.'

I say, 'Colston was a philanthropist, who gave money to build schools, hospitals and houses for the poor across Bristol.'

'Sorry to interrupt,' Ash says. 'Do you know if you do have time to extend the course by a couple of weeks?'

'I don't think I do,' I say.

Ash lowers his eyelids. He clenches his jaw.

I gesture at the image of Colston in his hand and say, 'Colston was also a slave trader. His company kidnapped around 100,000 people from West Africa. That's how he made a lot of his money.'

Ash rests the image on his lap.

'Should the statue be taken down?' I ask.

'If you allow it to stand there, then it's like you're saying it's OK to be inhumane,' Ash says.

'I've never understood that word,' Louis says. 'How can a human be inhumane? Anyway, they didn't believe slavery was wrong in those days.'

'Colston knew it was wrong,' Ash says.

'It's just like us in here. Two hundred years ago, the reasons people on the VP wing are inside wouldn't have even been a crime.'

'Look at all the money Colston gave away,' Ash says. 'He knew what he was doing was wrong.'

Louis says, 'So are we supposed to pretend people like him never existed? I tell you what, let's take down the statue! But on the condition that we take down every statue ever. Let he who is without sin cast the first stone. No, wait, forget that! Let's only remember everyone as the worst thing they've ever done.'

'That's not what I think we should do,' Ash says.

He picks up the image and looks at it.

'Get a chainsaw and cut the statue down the middle, so there's only half of him left,' he says.

Trust

> Those who trust us educate us.
> GEORGE ELIOT

A few weeks ago I started in a new prison and sat in a stuffy conference room with a dozen other people. We were listening to a security talk from a long-serving officer called Kern.

'Sometimes a resident asks you to do things for them,' he said. 'He'll ask you for today's paper, even though they know they're not allowed to have a copy of today's paper inside. If you say yes, then he'll ask you for a paper every day until you're used to bringing him things. He'll make you feel like you can trust him. Then he'll ask you to post a letter for him. You feel sorry for them and don't see any harm in it, so you do it. Then he asks you to bring in other things like money, drugs and phones. If you refuse, he'll threaten to report you for bringing newspapers in. Someone in this prison recently got fired when we found out she was topping up a prisoner's illegal mobile phone for them. That all started with harmless favours two years before. You might not think you're being groomed, but, remember, these guys have a lot of time on their hands. They can play the long game.'

He showed us an image of a twelve-inch makeshift knife handcrafted from steel with a handle wrapped in wire. Then he showed us a dozen more photos of grisly looking improvised weapons: a razor-blade toothbrush; a broomstick barbed with nails; a snooker ball in a sock. 'If you see a prisoner moving unnaturally, like they might be trying to conceal a weapon, tell someone.' He said that over the last ten years there had been more and more violence on the landing. A few months previously, he had to deal with one man jugging another – jugging is when someone boils their kettle, pours sugar inside and throws the water in someone's face. The hot sugar burns into their skin. Assaults on staff had also been on the rise. 'Never let anyone get too close to you,' he said. 'Guard your space.'

'Every object a prisoner has in their cell is somewhere to hide drugs,' he said. 'A tube of toothpaste or deodorant. In the middle of a packet of biscuits. In a slit cut in the sole of a trainer. In the binding of a book. Inside a pen they've nicked from education.

'But the latest new thing now is cybercrime,' he said. He told us about one man he worked with who used a smuggled-in smartphone to commit romantic fraud. He set up fake dating profiles with photos of handsome young men, searched for women in their fifties who said they were looking for happiness and manipulated them into transferring hundreds of pounds into his bank account. 'Last year a young lad here went on the library computer and hacked his way onto the internet. He was contacting witnesses and intimidating them.'

He concluded by saying, 'Keep your eyes open. Let them know early on you're not an idiot. Never trust a prisoner.'

If I treated the men in my class with as much fear and suspicion as Kern does, they would fold their arms, avoid making eye contact with me and keep their mouths closed. If they knew I was never going to trust them then why would they bother to be trustworthy? Kern's advice might be effective for keeping a particular type of order on the landing, but it's useless if you want to build relationships; it doesn't help people to grow.

I'm currently working in two prisons, one modern and the other old. The modern prison is cleaner and has wider corridors and bigger windows than the old one. But it also has sharper angles; the corners of each room are more square, whereas in the old prison the edges are rounded. I'm not sure which institution I find more severe. The modern prison looks like punishment in high resolution.

When I first started working in the modern prison, one of the teachers told me not to be afraid of the men. 'Once you get to know them, you realize that they have a heart of gold.' Two months later she got fired for bringing things in for a man. Sometimes teachers and officers react against each other like a pair of dysfunctional parents: the more severe and cynical security are, the more indulgent and romantic teachers become.

A few months ago, I was in the same prison teaching a class of mainstream prisoners and as the men were talking in pairs, a sweet-faced older man called Micky came up to me and showed me his wristwatch. 'My battery is running down,' he said. 'I put in an app asking for a new one weeks ago, but I've heard nothing.'

'They've probably lost it. I'd write another one,' I said.

'I'll just wait. Don't worry, I'm always waiting.'

'Write another app. You'll get your battery eventually.'

'I hope so, it was my brother's watch, before he died. You don't have a battery, do you?'

'I don't,' I said.

'Ha,' he said, as if acknowledging that the score was now 1-0 to me.

Today, I'm teaching in that prison and I have a student who is a similar age to me, called Gabriel. For the last few months he has been trying to write a prison memoir from his cell. Last week, he gave me the first ten pages to look at and said, 'I know I don't know lots of words like you do but I've got so many stories, Andy.' I read it but many of the words were illegible. Gabriel is dyslexic and uses bad handwriting to cover up his spelling mistakes. I'm also dyslexic and I do the same thing when I write by hand. I'm certain I wouldn't have got off the ground as a writer if I hadn't had a computer with a word processor and spellcheck. From the sentences I could make out in Gabriel's writing, he has a compelling story and some really fertile images. He writes every day, but I fear he's multiplying unreadable pages.

Today, at the end of a class, the men are trickling out. Gabriel stays behind to help me stack the chairs away. 'I can do it, Gabriel,' I say. But he keeps stacking the chairs until they are all away.

I pack my things in my bag and put my rucksack over my shoulder. Gabriel picks up his newspaper. It's over a week old and has a photo of Julian Assange on the front. I gesture towards the door. Gabriel stands still and says, 'Did you read my writing?'

'I did. I couldn't always make out the words,' I say.

'Neither can I. My handwriting is fucking awful.'

'Could you write it on a computer in the library?'

'I only get two hours a week in the library and that's taken away if there's a lockdown. What would really help me is if I had a laptop.'

In this prison, teachers can give men who are doing distance learning courses a personal laptop to use in their cells. But security must approve it first. Men cannot have a laptop if they are in for possessing images of child sexual abuse or cybercrime, or if security anticipate some other risk.

'Could you help me get one?' Gabriel asks.

I scan his face.

'It would really help me with my writing,' he says.

'I'll speak with one of the senior officers,' I say.

A female security officer outside the classroom puts her head in the door and says, 'We're gonna have to move you on now, sir.'

Ignoring the officer, Gabriel looks down at the picture of Assange on his newspaper. 'Where's Belmarsh?'

'Plumstead, near Woolwich,' I say.

He narrows his eyes at me.

'In south-east London,' I say.

'I know where Plumstead is,' he says, as if I have just spoken to him like he was an idiot. 'I passed through there many times, but I never saw a prison. But you never see them, do you? It wasn't until I came to this place last time that I knew it even existed. I drove past it every day when I dropped my kids off at school.'

'Sir, we are really going to have to go now,' the officer says.

'There are prisons everywhere,' Gabriel says, 'but they're always set back off the road, always walled-off by trees because they don't want the eyesore. Tall, thick bushes they use, so you can't see them.'

The officer walks into the class.

Gabriel goes on. 'Before I got recalled back to here, I was on a coach once and saw lots of green by the side of the road. I got this knot in my stomach.'

'Sir, I'm going to have to—'

Gabriel turns, pushes past the security officer and walks out through the door.

The officer rolls her eyes.

'It's like herding cats sometimes,' she says.

The next day, I'm in the old prison. I walk down the twos, past three officers who are searching someone's cell. The air is tinged with the smell of men living in confinement: the mixture of body odour, old mattresses, weed, floor cleaner, bad breath, and the emulsion that crumbling prisons are continually applying to the walls and steel-bar doors.

A minute later, I open my classroom door and the stench hits me. I go in and push open the windows that have been shut for the last twenty hours. The carpet is old and musty. The exposed foam on the seats has been sat on by the thousands of men passing through this institution. A small rat scuttles alongside the skirting board and disappears behind a cabinet. The fresh air comes in and as the smell dissipates, the room gets cooler.

A few minutes later, five or six men file in and each takes up a seat in the circle of chairs. I point them to the register and pen on my desk for them to sign their names. A man in his early thirties called Wesley comes in and says, 'Ready for another day in paradise.' His hair is flat on one side from where he has been sleeping. He wears a blue prison-issue T-shirt, but only on one arm, so the shirt rests diagonally across his body, showing his white vest underneath and his naked shoulder and bicep. He picks up my pen, looks at me and says, 'This is a nice pen.'

'Thanks,' I say.

'No, this is a nice pen.' He speaks with his head slightly ducked, his fist over his mouth as if he's MC'ing. 'People here don't get nice pens. This one's sharp as well. Bring a biro next time, unless you want your stuff to go missing. Why is it so cold in here? Close the windows, big man!'

I step towards the windows and say, 'As long as you don't mind the smell.' The men look at me blankly. They have adjusted to the smell. I pull the windows only half shut.

I go to the whiteboard and draw a frog and a scorpion next to a river. Next to my foot, a cockroach is squirming on its back. I kick it out of the way.

'Today I want to discuss a fa—'

A plane is flying low overhead and the drone of the engines becomes too loud to talk over. I rest my hands on my hips and pause. Under the noise, Wesley holds forth to two men on either side of him. His two friends nod at the words that are coming out of his mouth. The plane sound trails off and Wesley says, 'Isn't it!' He lowers his head, speaking into his fist. 'Every time I've had chicken in prison it's always the right leg.'

'How can you tell it's the right leg?' I ask.

Wesley stands up and brings his hands to his armpits to make wings and lifts one leg off the ground. 'What leg does a chicken stand on?'

I look at Wesley's feet. He has his left foot on the floor. 'Left leg?' I say.

'The right leg, the right one does all the work so it's got

less meat on it. That's the one they give to us. The left one goes to the NHS.'

'But how can you tell? Looking at a chicken leg, how can you tell if it's the left one or the right one?'

'If we complain, who is going to believe us?' Wesley says. His two mates beside him shake their heads at me.

'It's not that I don't believe you. It's that I just don't know myself how I could tell a left chicken leg from a right chicken leg,' I say.

'So you think they give a fuck if we eat healthy or not?'

'I'm trying to say how do you tell a left leg from a right one?'

'I like you, Andy, come on, you're not an idiot.'

'I'm vegetarian.'

The door opens. Ravel arrives late after coming from a legal visit. He has very short teeth that are all level, like they have been worn down from grinding. He takes his seat and complains that in the corners of the classroom there are two black mousetrap boxes with poison in them. This annoys him because men are not allowed bleach in their cells in case they use it for suicide. He has to put up with his cell smelling of his toilet.

'Even the vermin have more privileges than us,' Ravel says.

'What, did you think the screws was gonna use humane traps?' Wesley says.

I say, 'Today I want to discuss an old fable called the frog and the scorpion.'

Another plane is passing overhead.

I carry on. 'The story starts with the frog sitting in the grass, next to a river and watching the sun go down—'

The engines of the plane are too loud. I pause once more to wait for it to pass.

Wesley turns and talks to his two friends again. The sound of the engines fades out, and Wesley points up and says, 'One of them is gonna hit here one day.'

'Hundred per cent,' his friend mutters.

'Here?' I say.

Wesley says, 'If there's an engine failure and it has to crash land, where is the pilot instructed to? The nearest prison.'

I raise an eyebrow.

'The plane is going down. The pilot is looking out of his cockpit and sees the school, hospital, posh houses. Of course he's gonna go for the prison,' Wesley says.

I look at Ravel and he nods.

'They didn't tell me that when they offered me the job here,' I say.

'What headline do they want? "Kids dead in plane crash" or "Thieves and drug addicts dead in plane crash"?' Wesley says.

'Wouldn't all the people escape? Wouldn't they write "Thieves and drug addicts run free after plane crash"?'

Wesley tuts. 'I bet you believe the Americans didn't do 9/11 to themselves as well.'

'Back to the story,' I say.

'You do, don't you?'

'It's a story that has more than one interpretation.'

'You know I'm right, Andy,' Wesley says.

I tried to discuss conspiracy theories in here once before. I won't do it again. The men told me how we were all being controlled by malevolent forces and I tried to tell them that the world was more complicated than that. They all looked at each other and laughed.

'You reckon it was Al-Qaeda who did them towers?' says Wesley.

'The frog is sitting in the grass,' I say.

"What about the moon landings – real or fake?'

'He's by a river. The sun is going down.'

'The vape trails got into your brain, Andy.'

'The frog is in the grass and he's by a river and the sun is going down. Out of the grass comes a scorpion and it says to the frog that he needs to get home across the river but that he can't swim and that it will be dangerous for him to be out once it gets dark. He asks the frog if he can climb onto his back and for the frog to ferry him across the river.'

Wesley is finally listening.

'The frog says no,' I say. 'But the scorpion says he can guarantee the frog he won't sting him. "If I sting you in the water, then you'll drown. That means I'll drown too and we'll both die. I don't want to die. You can trust me, I promise. Please will you take me across the water?"'

Wesley narrows his eyes at me.

'The frog thinks about this. He thinks it makes sense and he agrees to ferry the scorpion across the river. The scorpion climbs onto the frog's back and the frog gets into the water and swims. Halfway across the water, the frog feels a terrible pain in his head.'

Wesley rolls his eyes.

I say, 'The pain travels down his back and through his body. His limbs feel heavy – the scorpion has stung him. As the frog is beginning to sink, he says, "Why did you do that? Now we'll both drown." The scorpion says, "I couldn't help it. It's my nature."'

'I thought you said that story had more than one

interpretation,' Wesley says. 'Frogs smoke weed. Is that the interpretation?'

'He should've,' says Ravel. 'At least then he'd be paranoid. The scorpion asks him for a ride and he'd be like, "Ohhh noooo! I don't have a good feeling about this, man."'

'OK, mushrooms then. Was he hallucinating?' Wesley says. 'Why would he take a scorpion on his back?'

'It's like when you go for parole and you try and persuade them you've changed. Then you get nicked again, and you're thinking it's their fault for letting me go last time,' Ravel says.

'Do you know what I wanna know?' says Wesley. 'Did the scorpion know the whole time that he was gonna sting him, or did he only know once he stung him? Like people in here – they say they're your friend and they aren't gonna rob you and then they rob you, but did they know they was gonna do that when they made friends with you or did they know they were only gonna rob you when they did it?'

'I know,' Ravel says. He comes to the board. I step away. He uses the side of his fist to rub out the river drawn on the board. 'If the river wasn't there, then this wouldn't happen. The environment was to blame.'

He sits back down and Wesley says, 'But there's always an environment. If there wasn't no environment, there wouldn't even be any animals.'

'But your jail friends who rob you, maybe they don't do that in a different environment.'

'They are called jail friends. It's in the name. This is their environment.'

A moment later, I say, 'What do other people think? Put your hand up if you think the frog is to blame?'

Another plane goes overhead.

All six men put their hand in the air or half in the air, except for Blake, a man who sits with his chair slightly set back in the circle. Blake has a bent nose and biceps so big that the fabric on his T-shirt is taut over them.

The noise of the plane passes.

'Blake, man, the frog is an idiot,' Wesley says.

'If you blame people for being kind, then what happens? No one wants to be kind any more,' says Blake.

'But the whole moral of the story is kindness has no place in nature,' Wesley says.

Ignoring Wesley, Blake says, 'If the scorpion knew his nature, then he was duty-bound to say to the frog what his nature was. It's like if you're a drug addict or you get put away for a domestic, the next time you get a girlfriend, you're duty-bound to tell her your nature.'

'How do you even know your nature is still gonna be your nature with this new girl?' Wesley says.

'Addiction is the nature of drug addicts.'

'You sound like one of the guvs. You see me – I'm in jail for a long time. Even if they let me out after half my sentence, I'm still doing another two years on top of the two I've already done. I got no time for this frog shit.'

Anger flickers in Blake's eyes. Wesley's mate nudges him and in a hushed voice he tells him how Blake is an IPP prisoner who has just been recalled four days after being released.

Wesley says, 'So you know what the real world is like then, Blake. If a man you didn't know says to you, "Oh, just come into my cell for a second," you don't go in, do you? If someone said, "Oh, thank you very much, I think I will," and then started complaining when the shanks came out and the hot water came out, you'd say to them, "Well, what the fuck did you expect?" Man is supposed to say, "Why do you want me to come into your cell? Tell you what, let's talk out here on the landing instead." The frog should be asking more questions.'

'Fifteen years ago, I would have blamed the frog,' says Blake. 'I'd have always taken the perpetrator's side. Back then I couldn't see that victims are victims.'

'Washed-ups always give the worst advice,' Wesley says.

'And you youngers always think the only way to survive the landing is to be a scorpion,' Blake says.

Wesley grins, tapping his fist against his mouth.

A few minutes later, Blake asks, 'Did the scorpion only realize what his nature was when he stung him? Or did he know all along?'

'We don't know,' I say. 'But what if he knew all along?'

'Then he's doubly responsible. My responsibility has increased the more self-aware I've become. I know it's my personality to abuse drugs. So when I do, I'm more accountable for it. I'm in here today for basically the same charge I went down for ten years ago. But I'm more guilty for this crime than I was for that.'

I hear a plane approaching overhead.

'Actually, Blake, now I think of it, I tell women I'm a liar all the time,' Wesley says as he laughs. 'I say, "One thing you should know about me is that I'm a really good liar." Do you know what they say to me? They say, "Thank you for being so honest." They say, "It's so good that you're being honest."'

He laughs again, but it's drowned out by the drone of the plane's engines.

★

I first met Lamar when I bumped into him on my lunch break in a vegan cafe around the corner from prison. He was wearing his prison officer uniform. He said he was a vegan so that he could be his best possible self whilst he was at work. In prison, he carried his keys in a special fabric pouch instead of the standard-issue leather one. He became an officer two years ago. He believed there was a more imaginative way of running prisons. He'd heard of exceptional institutions in Norway and Sweden where prisoners are treated like people and the reoffending rate is low, and therapeutic prisons in the UK like HMP Grendon that nurture agency and autonomy rather than destroy it. He wanted to be part of making that culture more widespread. But after a year into the job, Lamar was frustrated by how much of his day was spent herding men to and from their cells and keeping them locked up instead of developing nurturing relationships with them. His seniors didn't always support his ambition. On his night shifts, he sat in the office with an officer called Barber, who had worked in jails for two decades. Barber used to say to Lamar, 'Once a prisoner is twenty-two years of age, they're a lost cause. At nineteen or twenty, they can still be helped, but when they keep coming back at twenty-two and twenty-three, they will keep coming back again and again. We might as well keep them inside.' Lamar disagreed. 'If you don't give people the chance to change then they never will.' Barber sniggered. 'I was like you once. Wait until you've been in the job as long as I have.'

Perversely, I can relate to Barber's fatalism, only from the other side. When my brother was inside, I quickly became irritated by the mention of other countries that had more progressive ways of dealing with addiction and how they had less crime and fewer deaths. The days were more manageable if I told myself, 'It is what it is.' If I'd allowed myself to imagine a world where Jason could be getting the help he needed, I'd have been constantly furious. If another world was possible, I didn't want to know about it.

Last week, Lamar told me he was losing hope that he'd be able to influence the culture. He said that whenever a man sounds their buzzer during the night, there's one officer who mutters, 'I've got a bullet for each one of them.' I told Lamar that Oscar Wilde said that the most frightening thing about prison 'is not that it breaks one's heart – hearts are made to be broken – but that it turns one's heart to stone.'

'I worry that if I stay in the job I'll get used to prison and I'll go numb,' Lamar said. 'And I'm not even talking about the prisoners.'

The next day, I'm in the modern prison and at the end of my class, Gabriel comes up to me and says, 'I've been writing three pages a day for my book.'

'I forgot to ask about your laptop. I've been so busy,' I say.

'People always forget.'

'I'm sorry.'

'Why do people say they're sorry? I don't believe them. If they were really sorry they wouldn't have done it.'

'I'll ask today, Gabriel, I will.'

He turns and leaves without saying goodbye.

A few minutes later, in the corridor, I see Senior Officer Walsh, a woman in her early forties who has a utilitarian short haircut.

I tell her that Gabriel has been working hard on his book and has asked me to look into getting him a laptop.

Walsh looks me up and down. 'Can you come into my office, please,' she says.

We go into her office. It is cold and dank. She shuts the door. 'What did he ask you for?'

'Just what I told you now,' I say.

'The last time I gave someone a laptop, I later found out he was in debt on the wing.'

'And he sold it?'

'No. The men he owed would stop by his cell and use it to run their cybercrime business so that he carried all the liability, not them.'

'Is Gabriel in debt?'

'Now isn't the time to have more laptops floating about the wing.'

I rub my forehead with my fingers.

'Is this gentleman friendly to you?' Walsh asks.

'Yes, he always helps me pack up the class.'

'It's the ones who go out of their way to attract positive attention who are often the ones up to something.'

Walsh sits down at her desk to get on with her work.

I step to the door and open it. I turn around and say, 'He's genuinely working hard on his book.'

'I understand you want to help,' Walsh says. 'This place used to pull at my heartstrings too once upon a time. But I don't want us to get stung again.'

On my way out of the prison, I see Gabriel on the landing and tell him that I can't get him a laptop.

'I didn't expect anything different,' he says.

'Then why did you ask me to ask them?' I say.

He shrugs. 'It was a silly idea to try and write a book anyway.'

'You have a story. You should carry on.'

'Nobody can understand it. I'm only embarrassing myself.'

I wish I could knock down this building and build something more imaginative; a place that aimed to heal rather than merely contain people; where trusting and trustworthiness were nurtured; where the deprivation was not so extreme that people had to become 'manipulative' to meet their basic needs; where security were able to discriminate between people who are and aren't genuinely dangerous, instead of jadedly assuming that everyone is a scorpion in waiting.

But the building still stands.

The philosopher Susan Neiman says that when living in a problematic world you can easily fall into either defeatist resignation that things are what they are, or exhausting indignation that things are not what they should be. She says that to live well in the world you must learn to embrace how the world is and strive for how the world ought to be at the same time. We must live as much for the *is* as for the *ought*. If I am to stay aloft, I will have to find a way to work in prison whilst also wanting to tear it down.

The next morning I wake up to a message from Lamar. He tells me he has handed in his notice. He wants to work with a charity that helps kids who've been expelled from school, to help keep them out of jail. I'm happy to hear about his renewed sense of hope, but I know I'll find it harder to go into prison knowing that there will be one less person like him there.

A few hours later, I step into the old prison and my head starts to ache. I walk down the twos and see a pigeon is calmly perched on one of the thick pipes six inches from the ceiling. I stop to look at it. It must have flown over the wall and got into the building while a security door was open during free flow. It would have come through the gaps in the bars of the landing doors to get here.

An officer is walking past me. I point out the bird to him.

'Yeah, there's nothing you can do to keep them out,' he says. He walks on.

I go to my classroom and open the windows to get rid of the smell. There's a crisp, blue spring sky, but the north-facing classroom remains dingy, which I'm grateful for since bright light would only make my headache worse. Ravel and Wesley come in, talking about a fight they saw last night on the landing.

'I heard it before I saw it. He hit him clean,' Wesley says. 'It was like bang! You know when a punch makes you rethink your entire life? Man was like "um, um . . . um!"' Wesley strokes his chin to mimic someone deep in thought. Some of the others clap and laugh.

He goes to my desk, signs in and says, 'I told you, Andy, this is a nice pen. Are you desperate for it to get nicked or something.'

He drops the pen on the table. The rest of the men arrive. I close the door. A mouse scuttles along the skirting board.

I say, 'Dostoyevsky wrote a novel called *The Idiot*. It's about a character called Prince Myshkin, who is generous and open-hearted but everyone else in his world is corrupt and cynical. They ridicule, insult and threaten Myshkin, but he continues to see the good in them regardless. This makes the others mock him even more. They call him an idiot.'

'He's a mirror to the others, how corrupt they are. They're too afraid to look at their own reflection, so they gang up on him,' says Blake.

'This bloke is a prince, right? He's sheltered, doesn't live in the real world,' says Wesley.

I say, 'When Myshkin was younger, he was put before a firing squad. In the moment before the soldiers were due to fire, Myshkin saw the sunlight glinting off a church spire. It became so obvious to him that life was something beautiful. His execution was called off at the last moment. After that, he never wanted to forget how precious it was to be alive.'

'So if we want people to be nice then maybe we should put a gun in their face,' Wesley says.

My headache is getting worse.

Blake says, 'Myshkin's living with corruption on his doorstep, just like we do in here. But even though this place is full of criminals, I find it easier to be kind in here than I do on the outside.'

'Why?' I ask.

'When I was released last time, whenever I tried to be nice or do something good, people looked at me strange, wondering what I'm up to. No matter what I do on the outside, I'm just an ex-con. It's like I'm only allowed to be 2D in the world outside. But in here, when I give advice to someone doing their first jail, or I share my canteen, just a person helping another person. My kindness just is what it is. I'm allowed to exist in 3D when I'm in here.'

'What does that mean for Myshkin?' I say.

'Even though he knows the others are corrupt that makes him need to be good to them anyway, to hold on to himself,' Blake says.

'It's not good for him to be good in that world,' Wesley says. 'He's gonna get killed.'

'So would you tell Myshkin he needs to change?' I ask.

'If he was gonna change, he'd have done it by now,' Wesley says. 'Nobody ever really changes anyway. You can make people think you've changed, but that's different from actually changing. Me, when I arrive in jail, I deliberately act much badder than I usually am. They write it all down in my file. Then, after a month or two, I just act like myself. They write that in my file too. At the end of my sentence, when they read through my file, it looks like I've rehabilitated. But I'm still as bad as I ever was.'

'Oldest trick in the book,' Ravel says.

Blake says, 'I wouldn't tell Myshkin to change. I'd tell him to get out of that world.'

An hour later, the class ends and the men go back to their cells. I press my fingers into my scalp to try and release the tension in my head. I'm overwhelmed with the desire to be out of this prison. I grab my bag and head to the front gate.

I leave the prison, walk for fifteen minutes to a large park and sit on a bench under a tree. In the distance, parakeets cruise from one tree to another. They are lime green but look silver silhouetted against the light of the early evening. There's a long breeze, the poplar trees above me sway and the rustling leaves make a white noise. My headache starts to fade.

I feel spots of water on my arms and hands. A gentle rain falls and brings out the woody smell of the trees and the earthy mud. But I can also smell something musty. The smell of the prison is on my clothes.

Two months on, I notice myself becoming more numb to prison. Last week, two prison officers started fighting each other on the landing and security had to lock down the wings while they coped with it. I was mostly annoyed that I wouldn't be able to use the photocopier. Yet I also find myself becoming overly frustrated by small things, like when I don't have enough pens for the men or when I'm trying to use a knackered set of keys.

I haven't seen Gabriel for a few weeks, but today another teacher at work tells me that he has started writing his book again.

Salvation

> Speech will be the business of men.
> TELEMACHUS

In 2018, a man called Tyrone Givans hanged himself in his cell after spending three weeks on remand. An inquest found that Givans had spent almost a month in prison without his hearing aid. The security officers who worked with him hadn't realized he was profoundly deaf. They said he seemed to understand what they were saying as long as they spoke slowly.

This Monday morning, I'm teaching a group of mainstream prisoners. One of my students in the circle, Glennton, has a hearing aid. There are also a few men in their early twenties. The group is incredibly loud. They only had two hours out of their cells since Friday dinner time. I can hear their pent-up energy in the volume of their voices.

I give them ten minutes to decompress. Then I tell the class, 'Plato tells the story of a man called Gyges who finds a ring of invisibility. Once Gyges puts on the ring, he can kill, steal and do anything without anyone finding out.'

'Unless they spin his cell,' Glennton says.

'Plato asks, would there be any reason for Gyges to be good?' I say.

'Females,' Glennton says.

I raise one eyebrow.

Glennton goes on. 'When I was begging, I'd see three lads out together and I knew that I wasn't going to get any money from them. If I did, they'd only give me something after making me the butt of their joke first. But if I saw a man out with a woman – then things were different. She has a shopping bag from where he's just bought her something. They're giving off honeymoon vibes. I go up and ask him for money. Now he has the chance to show that he's kind and that he's got cash to give away. The joke of it is, I'd say thank you to him, but I'm helping him win the woman. Without me, he's spending his Saturday night as one of those three lads. He should be thanking me. I'm his golden ticket.'

'So Gyges should be good if women can see him?' I ask.

'Look at this place, Andy. All the female teachers, nurses, security, drug workers. Take them out of here and do you think men are gonna behave better or worse?'

There's the sound of voices from outside in the yard. Three of the younger men in my class run over to the window. They bang the glass. 'I see you! I said I can fucking see you!' one of them shouts.

I stand behind them and look over their heads. On the other side of an internal wall, VPs are being transported back to their wing.

'I'm gonna cut your dick off, I swear,' one of the boys shouts.

'Gentlemen,' I say.

'My last jail, I was on the servery. I spat in their food every day.'

'Can we get back to Plato?' I say.

Glennton turns down his hearing aid.

The young men stay at the window, shouting threats of torture until the VPs are out of sight. I ask the boys to sit back in the circle, but they're too excited. The three of them have a quick-fire exchange of stories about prison fights.

Ten minutes later, I finally get them to sit down. They carry on discussing the ring of invisibility with residual violence in their voices.

An hour later, I leave the prison and take out my phone from my locker. I have a missed call from my brother. I call him back, but there's no answer.

A few hours later, I receive an email to confirm that I'm cleared to do a few classes in a women's prison next month. It comes as a relief. I hadn't anticipated how much I'd encounter my convoluted feelings of inherited guilt by working with men in prison. I'm hoping that working with women inside won't be as triggering.

The next morning, I arrive at the security gate of a men's prison. I take off my shoes and belt and put them into a tray for inspection. A female officer with peroxide white hair is calling out 'Next!' to people standing in the line ready to pass through a security scanner. I join the queue. One of the governors comes in and stands behind me. He takes off his shoes and belt and joins the line. He has yellow and pink zigzags on the tips of his socks. We chat for a few minutes and I tell him I'm due to start teaching in a women's prison.

'The one and only day I worked in a women's prison, I left feeling so awful about myself for being a man,' the governor says. 'You hear all of these women's stories. They're all there because of some bloke.'

'Next!' the officer calls.

'Like what?' I ask the governor.

'I'd say well over half of them were victims of domestic

violence. Often, they were the ones inside for something they'd done to support their boyfriend's drug habit. So many of them had been trafficked or sold into sex work as teenagers. One day there. That was enough for me. I drove home that night feeling disgusted with myself for belonging to the male sex.'

'Next!' the officer calls.

'I'm there a few days,' I say to the governor.

'Excuse me, sir!' says the officer, raising her voice at me. 'You're next!'

I step into the scanner.

I was six years old. My father was topless on the couch and watching the TV. He had swirls of dark hair on his chest and shoulders and he was smoking filter tips and drinking beer from a can. I was sitting on the floor between him and the telly. An advert came on appealing for donations to help starving children. The shape of their bones showed through their skin. My father removed the lid off a tin of chocolates on the coffee table next to him, took out a chocolate and threw it at the screen.

I turned and gave him a desperate look. He laughed out loud. I wanted to say 'Don't,' but the words were trapped inside me. He had another swig of his beer, took another chocolate out of the tin and threw it again. It went past my head and made a 'dink' sound as it hit the glass of the screen.

I always felt nervous around my dad. He was so unpredictable. If we were in the car and someone in the vehicle behind beeped their horn at him, he might stop the car, get out and holler abuse in the driver's face. Or he might just look in his mirror, swear and carry on driving.

But there were times when I knew what to expect. On Sunday afternoons before we went to the pub, he and I would wait in the living room while Mum got dressed and put on her make-up. During that period, we'd have police or bailiffs knocking on our door. The neighbours would look out their windows. Mum never left the house looking anything other than perfect.

Dad and I waited for her to get ready, me trying to avoid his eye. Eventually, she'd come downstairs wearing lipstick, smelling of perfume, and ask him if she looked OK.

'Andrew, what is she?' he would say.

I'd look up at him, trying not to let him see how afraid I was.

'She's a tart,' I'd say.

'That's right. She's a tart,' he'd say.

Mum rolled her eyes.

I can't recall when my dad first trained me in that hateful little ritual. I just remember when he said, 'Andrew, what is she?' I knew that if I said, 'She's a tart,' then he would say, 'That's right. She's a tart.'

My colleague Patricia has taught in this prison for two decades. She is heavyset, has a working-class northern accent and is something of a mother figure to repeat offenders. I've seen men go to her for marriage advice or to show her the drawing they have done on the front of their children's birthday card. They practically sit on her knee and cry whilst other men sulk that Patricia's attention is going to someone else. If I were to say the things that she says to them, I would get my nose broken. She says things like: 'If you don't shut your trap, I will shut it for you!' or 'I want you all out of the room for the next ten minutes. The room stinks and I need you lot gone so I can breathe again.' The men almost always go 'He-he-he,' like little boys.

A few months ago, she came into my class and wrote at the top of my whiteboard: 'Don't forget International Men's Day on Wednesday.'

Glennton said, 'Why is there an International Men's Day? Ain't it women who've had everything shit for ages?'

'You can spend International Men's Day cleaning my classroom then,' Patricia said.

'Actually, it's quite hard being a man, now that I think of it,' Glennton said.

'You wouldn't clean it properly anyway. Men never do.'

An Albanian called Berat said, 'In this country, first is woman, then the child, then the dog. At the bottom is the man.'

'Which one are you: the dog or the child?' Patricia said.

'He-he-he,' Berat tittered.

In 2010, a twenty-eight-year-old female prison officer was jailed for having an intimate relationship with a man who was inside for raping and organizing an acid attack on his ex-girlfriend. Stories like that linger in prison for a long time and create no-win situations for female officers working with the men.

Last year, I worked with an officer in her thirties called Ms Olufemi. She kept a strict emotional distance when talking to the men. She worried that if she was seen to be too caring, then rumours would circulate that she was sleeping with one of them. Even though she'd know it wasn't true, it'd still be embarrassing and undermining of her authority. One day Ms

Olufemi came into work to find a mentally ill man had drawn a picture of her with huge breasts on his pillow. He was walking around the landing, cuddling it.

She went from being emotionally distant to demonstrably curt with the men. A few weeks ago, I saw a man on the landing asking Ms Olufemi if she could increase his privileges. He wanted more visiting time with his family.

'I can't just give it to you because you ask for it,' she said.

'Please, miss. You're not a cruel person, I know you're not,' the man said.

'No,' she said.

He tutted. 'Oh please, miss!'

'Sorry, no.'

'Fucking cold bitch,' he said and stormed off.

I travel to a rural prison a few hundred miles from London to teach a one-off workshop. I arrive early and sit on a bench in the car park and try calling my brother. The phone rings, but he doesn't answer.

Twenty minutes later, in the library, the class is underway. The atmosphere is tense. Nobody opens up. When people do talk, they share their ideas with me, but not with each other. I invite them to debate with one another, but they just keep talking directly to me. Hardly anyone voices disagreement. They say things like, 'It just depends on your opinion, I suppose.' The conversation keeps fizzling out into silence.

An hour later, the class ends and the men leave. A cheerful-looking librarian helps me stack the chairs in the corner of the room.

'How did it go?' he asks.

'The discussion never caught fire,' I say.

'That's good,' he says. He tells me that the group was half mainstream prisoners and half VPs.

'I wish they'd talked to each other,' I say.

'At least it wasn't a bloodbath,' he says.

Twenty minutes later, I leave the prison, take my phone from my locker and see my brother has tried to call me back. I call him back, but there's no answer.

I'm at my friend Chloe's dinner party. Opposite me sits a doctor called Paul, elegantly dressed in black. I tell him what I do and he says to me, 'So your dad was in prison and you teach in prison. Are you trying to save these men you teach?'

'Not really,' I say.

In my class the next day, I wear an ironed shirt, something I've not done in years. Rather than do the register by sight I call it out, like a professional would. I stop calling my students 'fellas' and start referring to them as 'gentlemen'. I interrupt students who interrupt other students and tell them that they must not interrupt. 'You're in the mood, aren't you?' one says to me.

In the afternoon, walking home, I listen to loud sweary music on my earphones, and in my head I re-enact a fantasy version of my conversation with Paul.

'Are you trying to save these men you teach?' says fantasy Paul.

'What did your parents do, Paul?' I reply.

'They were both doctors.'

'And you're a doctor too. How funny that you don't pathologize that type of inheritance.'

Fantasy Paul doesn't know what to say back. He looks six

inches shorter. Chloe offers me a second slice of cake. I eat it and gulp a mouthful of lapsang souchong.

Nobody wants to talk to fantasy Paul any more and he gets his coat to leave, but I put my arm around him and tell him to come and have a drink with me on the patio. Outside, under the stars, I tell him, 'It's not a matter of saving anyone, but a matter of what knowledge has been planted in your system. You don't get to decide what you have to digest.'

'I'm so grateful you taught me all this,' fantasy Paul says. He looks shy now, almost like a child.

The following week, I go to Chloe's house for Friday night drinks and Paul is sitting on the sofa. I pick the seat furthest away from him.

My mum enjoyed art lessons when she was a kid but found the rest of school to be like 'doing time'. The classrooms were chaotic. The police were often called in to stop fights. In class, she felt like the teachers were going through the motions with the girls, teaching them things, but as if it was something they didn't need to know. They were expected to become wives. She left school when she was fifteen to work on a market stall. Making money was much more thrilling than trying to survive the school day. Soon after, she got a job window dressing on the high street. It reminded her of those moments when she was drawing or painting at school. She married at seventeen. Throughout her twenties and thirties, she wished she could paint, read, learn to speak a foreign language. But she didn't have the time. Dad was often unemployed. He'd occasionally have jobs, but after a few weeks he'd fall out with someone and leave. Mum had to earn the money. If she ever did sit down on the sofa and read a book, Dad would have got jealous.

When I was a child, on Saturdays, Dad would go to the bookies and Mum and I would get in the car and go for a 'me and you day' in town. The moment we turned the corner at the end of our street, Mum became more relaxed. In town, we went into clothes shops and she'd try on dresses and shoes. There were things she couldn't afford, but she tried them on anyway just to look in the mirror and see what she looked like. One time we went into an art supplies shop and she picked up different shades of green paint off the shelf – lime, jade, emerald. 'When you're older,' she said, 'make sure you don't marry until you're over thirty.' She put the paints back.

We'd go to McDonald's. When we finished our food I'd say, 'Do we have to go home?'

'I know, mate. I'm dreading it too,' she'd say.

To cheer her up, I did my impression of Dad. I pretended I was driving and put on a Scouse accent, threatening the imaginary driver next to me that I'd knock him out. Mum would cry with laughter and then look around to make sure Dad wasn't behind her.

Today, Mum has a canvas she painted hanging in her living room. It's a naive landscape of green and blue mountains. Ten years ago, she bought herself an English to Greek dictionary to find the words for things like fridge, chair, curtains – *psygeío, karékla, kourtínes*. Today, she can talk in broken sentences about history, ruins and gods. Sometimes I buy two copies of a novel and send one to her so we can read them together. When we talk about it on the phone, she is always fifty pages ahead of me. After Mum separated from my dad, she wanted to move on as much as possible. She looks at me – how my life is free from violence, drugs, crime and chaos – and she says that everything that happened in the past was worth it, as if my freedom was her salvation. That's why she feels bad when I tell her that I still carry a sense of inherited guilt. I try to tell her that it's not her fault.

One evening when I was seven, I was at home with only Dad. He was sat in his armchair, watching the news and chain-smoking. I sat on the opposite corner of the room to him, playing with toys. Mum was out doing overtime at work.

It was past eight o'clock and Dad hadn't fed me. Mum came home. I told her I was hungry. She sat down on the sofa and told me she needed to rest for two minutes before she could cook.

Dad started an argument with Mum. He hated her working overtime because that meant she'd have spent a few extra hours with her colleague Mark. I did what I always did when they started rowing and switched the TV channel from the news to something I wanted to watch. I knew Dad wouldn't notice for ages.

An hour or so later, my face felt hot and my eyelids were heavy. My stomach was hurting with hunger, but my parents were still arguing.

'Mum, you said you'd cook,' I said.

'I will, I promise,' she said.

'Did I say you could change the channel?' Dad said to me. I froze.

'Put the news back on!' he said.

'The news has finished,' I said.

'Do as I fucking tell you,' he said.

My shoulders tensed up towards my ears. 'Mum, I'm hungry. Tart.'

'Fucking come over here now,' Dad said.

I walked over and stood between his legs. He sat forward in his chair, so his face was two inches from mine. He had tobacco stains in the grooves of his teeth. My legs trembled.

'What the fuck did you say?' he said.

I knew if I tried to speak, I'd start crying, so I kept my mouth shut.

'If you ever talk to your mother that way again, I'll fucking kill you. Do you understand?'

The morning before I'm due to start teaching in the women's prison, I stand in front of my bedroom mirror. I look at the left side of my face and then turn to look at the right side. I look like my father today. I've started to resemble him more since I turned thirty. I fluff up my hair to see if it changes the shape of my face, but I still look like him. It's in my forehead and my jaw. The executioner tells me there's nothing I can do to change it.

Throughout the morning, I think of my dad. I remember the time he bought me my first bicycle. I get a lot of joy from cycling today. I picture his yellowed fingertips. He smoked sixty cigarettes a day. I think of how unhappy he must have been to need to smoke that much. I imagine him as he might be today, an old man, frail and harmless. I search my mind for a story I can tell about him that might inspire kindness or pity. I did the same yesterday when I was cooking and the day before when I was trying to read a book. Throughout the twenty years since I decided to end contact with my dad, there is always a point in the day when I try to save him.

*

A few hours later, I'm having lunch with Patricia in the staff mess. She tells me about a twenty-four-year-old drama teacher called Divika, who has been coming into the prison once a week to run a course with the men.

'It's like she doesn't even try and hide it,' Patricia says. 'She wears a silk blouse and slinks around the room like some kind of cat. On her first day, she took a special liking to Rudge.'

Rudge has a scar down one side of his face. He's in the ninth year of his sentence.

'She sat next to him in the circle for the first few weeks, always touching his arm when she spoke,' Patricia says.

'Beauty and the Beast,' I say.

'Well, Rudge had seen this kind of thing all too many times before. The amorous part of him switched off a few years into his sentence. She wasn't getting a response out of him. After a few weeks, she moved places and sat next to Gareth instead.'

Gareth's teeth were severely decayed in the years of his heroin addiction and he was halfway through a dental plan to rebuild them when he got recalled to prison. Now he smiles with his lips pursed together. Keen to resist the drug culture on the landing, he converted to Islam a few months ago. He doesn't fully agree with the Imam's thing about no sex before marriage, but he thought that being in prison would make that academic anyway.

According to Patricia, Divika came in, her feminine presence perfuming the air, and gave Gareth a big hug at the end of each class. Gareth would just stand there, her hair in his face. He tried not to touch her but not to push her away either. The other men in the room put their hands over their mouths to muffle their laughter.

★

After lunch with Patricia, I'm walking down the landing. Men are banging on the doors. A high-pitch alarm rings out. There's the sound of staff radios, shouting, keys. Every noise echoes off the metal or concrete interior. I make out a man wailing from inside his cell, but I cannot tell if he is above or in front of me. His door could be two or ten metres away. Every sound is levelled in the cacophony. On the cell door to my left, I see a mouth and nose through the vertical slit of Perspex. A man is attempting to shout a message to the cell to my right, where a man places his ear against the slit. I cannot make out what they are saying to each other because of the din, but the man on my right puts his thumb up to the one on the left. Their hearing is more adjusted to this place than mine.

I get to my classroom. There's a faded poster on the wall just above my desk. It has an image of a woman being shouted at by a man. Below, it says, 'Next time you are about to abuse a female member of staff, remember, she is someone's SISTER, MOTHER, DAUGHTER.'

The poster makes me think of Helen, a colleague I co-taught with at a men's high-security prison last year. She was a petite woman with strawberry-blonde hair and an oval face. Some of the men would gawp at her with impossible lechery, others were dismissive, habitually correcting her or talking on as if she hadn't said anything, but at the end of the day, Helen and I would leave the prison and we'd take the train home and she would complain about how undermining it was when a lifer called Pawel picked out the best chair in the room for Helen each week. She asked him not to, but he kept doing it. Pawel called Helen 'Miss', despite her asking to be called Helen. When the other men interrupted her, Pawel stepped in and said, 'Have some respect. How would you feel if she was your sister?' Frustrated, Helen told him it wasn't necessary for him to intervene, but Pawel never stood down from his position.

After several weeks of this, Helen and I were talking about it on the train home together. She looked worn down.

'He just won't listen to what I'm saying,' Helen said.

'You're his salvation. He has to protect you from the other men to prove that he's not like them,' I said.

Helen shuddered.

An officer in the corridor shouts, 'Free flow.' I set my rucksack down on my desk to block out the poster. I go into the corridor and wait for the men to come.

A few minutes later, Mervin arrives. He has thin dreadlocks and a beard down to his chest. We bump fists and he stands, side-on to me, lamenting the most recent poor performance of his football club, Manchester United. An officer standing two metres away is also a United fan and joins in, complaining about the club's lack of decent signings. The three of us have a conversation. When Mervin talks to me, he looks me in the eye. But when he responds to the officer, he looks up at the ceiling.

A man called Marlon walks into the corridor. There's a flat patch of scar tissue where the tip of his nose should be. A decade ago, some drug dealers used a razor blade to claim the debt Marlon owed them in skin. Today, he wears a green T-shirt with the word 'Listener' on the back to indicate that he's an appointed Samaritan, available to give emotional support to men on the landing. When last month I chatted to him on the wing he told me how the work had changed him. 'When I was younger I would have thought of this kind of thing as soft. But I get as much listening to them as they do having someone to talk to. We both get to be actual people for a change.' We said goodbye and I watched him walking back down the landing. He still moved with a macho gait in his walk. I thought of how difficult it must be to grow and to survive in this place at the same time. Marlon can open his heart, but he still has to protect his body.

Gareth and a few more men arrive. We go into the class and sit around the table. Mervin and Marlon are laughing about an advert that was on TV when they were kids. It gave children a phone number they could call if their parents had beat them.

'My dad told me I was allowed to call that number if I wanted, and when the person came around, he'd slap me up and then slap them up in front of me,' Marlon says.

'I remember those ads. My dad burst out laughing when they came on,' says Mervin.

The two men laugh and high-five each other.

It's not uncommon in prison to hear men inside talking with bravado about their fathers' violence towards them when they were children. Their stories always make me flinch, but what is just as toe-curling is imagining that some of these fathers might have been anticipating that their boys would one day have to survive prison, that the blows were struck to prepare the child for a world where punishment is unfair.

Inside, I hear so many stories of boys who inhaled the toxicity from their violent dads and have grown up to become violent men themselves. When I was around my dad, it was like I was always holding my breath. To make sure I didn't repeat the cycle, I unconsciously appointed the executioner to watch over me. It has stopped me from going to prison, but it hasn't made me free.

I stand in front of the group, ready to start. But the men carry on talking. They're complaining about things. The portion sizes of the food. The officers who look at you like shit. The officers that pretend to be nice to you but won't do anything for you. An application that they've written four times with no reply and been told to write again. The fact they haven't had a transfer. The fact they are being transferred when they don't want to be. The water pressure of the showers. Not getting paid for their job sewing prison-issue boxer shorts. Not being able to get a job sewing prison-issue boxer shorts.

In the past, I used to believe I could simply wait out the complaining. I'd give the men five minutes to get their gripes off their chest. Once the noise had fizzled out, I could get on with the lesson. But there are an endless amount of things to be upset about in here and the men have little power to change any of them. The drone of complaining never fizzles out by itself.

'Can you finish your conversations, please,' I say.

They carry on. They complain about the queue for the barber. How prison-issue coats aren't thick enough to keep you warm out on the yard. How they still don't have the prison-issue coat they ordered. The queue for the phone. The nurse who only gives you a tiny cup of water with your morning medication and how you have to choke back your saliva to swallow your pills.

★

A minute later, I ask the men again for their attention. A few of them look at me. A couple are mid-complaint and have to finish what they are saying.

A few moments later, the room is finally quiet.

'Norman Mailer tells a story: two men pass each other on the street and say good morning. One of them loses,' I say.

Everyone in the room laughs.

I continue, 'Some philosophers say masculinity is an identity achieved through dominance. In order for me to be a man, somebody else has to lose. That often has to be women or children. Sometimes other men too.'

'But there are good men and there are bad men,' Marlon says.

I say, 'The feminist writer bell hooks says the idea of the good man is sexist. So is the idea of a good woman.'

'How do you be good then?' Marlon says.

'hooks says men should focus on trying to be a good person instead.'

'Being in prison, I don't care if I'm a good person,' Marlon says, 'but I feel bad about not being a good man. When I'm on the phone to my ex and I hear my little girl has a teacher who doesn't like her and I can't go and sort it out because I'm in here, or when my mum needs something and I can't provide for her, I feel like shit.'

'hooks don't even make sense. How can you stop being a good man? If you're a man you're a man,' Mervin says.

I put an A3-size picture of Malcolm X in the middle of the table. X wears a suit and is talking behind a podium.

'hooks says that over the course of his life, Malcolm X stopped worrying about being a good man. He became more focused on what kind of person he was instead,' I say.

'I saw a film about him,' Marlon says.

'I read his whole book,' Mervin says.

I say, 'Malcom X was a man of transformations. When he went to prison at twenty-one for robbery, he was illiterate. But he educated himself inside and when he was released, he became one of the Nation of Islam's most compelling voices. Also, he changed his name twice. At one point he was a black separatist but changed his mind after he met white Muslims at Mecca.'

'Didn't he copy out the whole dictionary?' Marlon says.

'Every single page. In his cell. It's like he was always reaching for the next thing. He became a criminal to get away from poverty, then he joined the Nation to get away from crime, then left the Nation for the next thing,' Mervin says.

'hooks says X was halfway through another transformation when he got assassinated,' I say. 'In some of his earlier speeches, X talks about how men are strong by nature and women are weak by nature. He thinks women don't have what it takes to lead in the struggle for black emancipation. He advises men to control women if they want their respect.'

'He grew up with no dad, didn't he? Loads of men in here only had their mums growing up. But so many of them are misogynistic though,' Marlon says.

'Blame the one who is still there, isn't it?' Mervin says.

Marlon says, 'People here don't even understand what sexism means. If a rapist moves onto their landing, they'll join the line of men queuing outside his cell. But when you see those same men walking around the landing—'

'Hands on their balls!' Mervin says.

'Every time, hands down the front of their trousers touching their balls, with female staff walking around. They'll mash up a rapist, but they don't get they're acting like one,' Marlon says.

'These are the same men chatting about how they deal drugs to pay their mum's bills. Bullshit! They're wearing Nike exclusives and a Rolex, but their mum is still shopping at Iceland,' Mervin says.

'My grandma would kill me if she knew my trainers came from drug money,' Marlon says.

'Mine would kill me if I went in her house with my trainers on,' Mervin says.

I bring the conversation back to Malcolm X. 'Later in his life, when he left the Nation of Islam, he said, "I feel like a man who has been asleep and someone under someone else's control. Now I think with my own mind." He met impressive female activists like Fannie Lou Hamer and Shirley Graham Du Bois. He acknowledged that women played an equal role to men in the struggle and said that in many cases, women had made a greater contribution than many men. He went from being threatened by how women might emasculate him by not showing him respect to admiring the intelligence and strength of certain women.'

The room goes quiet. A few of the men look at me sceptically.

I carry on. 'Imagine if X had lived and kept maturing, being less hung up on being a man. What could he have become? How else might he have evolved in his relationship to women?'

Marlon folds his arms. Mervin rolls his pen between his finger and thumb. I hear the sound of an officer's radio going off coming from the corridor.

'What do you fellas think?' I ask.

'When I see a hot security officer, I deliberately just say nothing,' Mervin says. 'Don't start a conversation unless you absolutely have to. Don't allow for any confusion.'

Marlon grunts in agreement. 'You can't help but feel sexual about women in here because you're so starved of sexual contact. You've got your prison goggles on. Every woman looks beautiful.'

'It's better not to engage with them. They already think we're bad people anyway. They might accuse me of something,' Mervin says.

'Or you don't want to end up like Gareth,' Marlon says.

The men jeer and laugh. Gareth looks embarrassed.

'Do you know what pissed me off most about all that?' Gareth says. 'When I was at school, all the posh girls weren't interested in me because I had a rep as a roadman, so I only went out with girls from my estate who wanted a bad boy. But now I'm thirty and in jail, all the girls on my estate have kids and only want someone who can provide and be responsible, but the middle-class girls love me. Where was they when I was sixteen?'

'I don't say anything to them. Especially the posh ones,' Mervin says.

Mervin says, 'Last week, on the landing, there was a young female officer outside a man's open cell keeping watch on him because he'd tried to commit suicide. You didn't even need to look at her to know she was hot.'

'You could tell by how fresh all the men looked on the landing that day,' Marlon says.

'Men was strutting up and down the landing past her,'

Mervin says. 'Men who don't even shave when their wives visit were looking good. And the trainers – oh my god, I saw Louis Vuittons I didn't even know existed.'

'Men were stopping and chatting to her, asking if the man on watch was OK and showing her their sleeve tattoos,' Marlon says.

'In the end, the guy on suicide watch was moaning to her, "You're not here to look after them. You're supposed to be looking after me."'

'I stand with my back to her whenever I see her.'

'I do exactly the same. Don't get me wrong, I don't have anything against her personally. I just want to keep things simple,' Mervin says.

'Don't get pulled in,' Marlon says.

'Don't look like a fool,' Mervin says.

Both men lean back in their chairs and fold their arms.

I pick the image of Malcolm X up from the table and hold it up. I say, 'So if he was here today, he'd say nothing?'

'It's the safest option,' Marlon says.

'Safest option, yeah,' Mervin says.

Thirty minutes later, I'm waiting at the bus stop outside the prison. I feel deflated. I wish the men could have given me something more than 'Say nothing.' Chloe messages to invite me to join her for drinks this evening. The bus to take me to hers pulls over next to me. I wave it on. Paul will probably be at Chloe's. I imagine if I told him about the class I ran today, he'd pick up his glass of wine with one of his long clean hands, sip from it and then smugly set it back on the table.

My bus arrives and I get on it. I stand, holding on to the pole above my head. To my left sits a little boy in school uniform. He is next to his dad, who is on his phone looking at girls on Instagram. The boy is playing with two small Lego men, pretending they are fighting each other.

A few weeks after the night my dad told me off for calling Mum a tart, I was sat in the back seat of our car playing with an action figure. Dad was driving and Mum was in the passenger seat. We were going out to the pub. Mum took out her lipstick and make-up mirror.

Dad looked in his windscreen mirror and said, 'Andrew, what is she?'

I squeezed the action figure, flying it in loops.

'What is she, Andrew?' he said.

I kept flying the figure around.

'He's in his own world. He can't hear you,' Mum said.

I travel on the bus for fifteen minutes. I press the stop button for the bus driver to pull over at the next stop. The little boy drops one of his Lego men near my foot. His dad, still swiping on his phone, doesn't notice. I pick it up and pass it to the child.

In the evening, I'm in the shower. I wash my hair and scrub my face. After I'm clean, I stand under the stream of water for several minutes.

I don't sincerely want to save my dad. I want to save myself. I want to make him less bad, so I don't have to inherit his badness. But all the while, I'm trapped within the logic of inherited guilt: if Dad is bad, I am bad. If I am to think of myself as a decent person, Dad must have also been decent. I can't separate myself from him.

I step out of the shower and brush my teeth in front of the mirror. I look exhausted.

I go into my bedroom and pack my rucksack with books and ID ready for going to the women's prison in the morning. I double-check the bag to make sure a kilo of heroin or a nine-inch kitchen knife isn't inside it.

I sit on the end of my bed, my overhead light still on. I hear the sound of the last train pulling out of the station behind my flat. I pick up my phone and call my brother.

He answers. 'Bruv,' he says. 'It's late. Are you OK?'

'I just wanted to hear your voice.'

Forgetting

Of all our sorrows, memory is the worst.
                              MARY BOYKIN CHESNUT

The women's prison used to be a men's jail, but when the female prison population got bigger, the government moved the men, replaced the urinals with cubicles and brought the women in. There are doors made of iron bars, but some of the corridors are painted in light pink. In the security room in one of the men's institutions I work in, there are framed images of the prison Alsatians. Throughout the women's prison, there are several canvas photos of the same white kitten. It has emerald-green eyes and oversized ears. On one image, it's playing with string. In another, it's being cupped in a human hand.

The women's prison is twice the size of the men's prison I was in last week, yet it only holds about a quarter of the number of people. It's less punishing on the senses: there is more green space and more light on account of the absence of towering buildings. I can smell grass and, unlike in men's prisons, when I walk through the grounds, strangers say hello to me.

When my boss Hannah heard I'd be working in a women's prison, she grinned and said, 'I bet they'll all want to do philosophy with Mr West.' In my first class, fifteen women squeezed into the classroom. Today, for the second class, only four have shown up.

Agnes, a woman with short spikey grey hair, reaches into her tote bag, takes out two small-sized Mars bars and holds them out to me.

'But they're yours,' I say.

'And I want you to have them,' she says, pushing the Mars bars up towards me again.

An officer passing through the room looks over at us. The prison rules say staff are not permitted to accept gifts from the women. Security are worried about things like grooming, inappropriate relationships or that staff could smuggle things out for the women.

'I'm sorry, Agnes.'

She drops her hand on her lap. 'Who makes these fucking rules? – excuse my language. It's just a fucking Mars bar.'

She puts the chocolates back in her bag. The officer leaves the room.

A Romanian woman called Sofia says, 'Can we just start?' She is wearing a royal blue blouse that would be fit to wear for a job interview. She has been in prison for over ten years but somehow still gets frustrated when things drag. Last week, she told me that sometimes the officers unlock her door on time in the morning, but sometimes they open it twenty minutes or an hour late. Ignoring the clock, she sets to an intense workout of press-ups, bicycle crunches, Russian twists, etc. 'When they unlock my door, they're not going to see me sitting there waiting,' she said to me. 'They're gonna see me flying.'

I get the lesson underway. I talk about memory and identity for a few minutes and then ask, 'If you lost your memory, would you still be the same person?'

'I think you become more you as you get older,' a woman called Dita says. She's wearing sunglasses because she didn't have time to use make-up to cover the bags under her eyes this morning.

'Like, I'm becoming more myself since I came here,' she says.

'Here?' I say.

'This is me-time.'

Before coming here, some of these women were sleeping rough, or they'd been a parent since they were fifteen, or were doing sex work and being given a ten per cent cut of the money by their pimps.

There is a knock at the door. I open it and eight of my students file in. They are laughing and chatting. They say they are late because one of their friends was being released and they went to the gate to say goodbye to her.

They each take their seat in the circle of chairs. Some of them sit so close to each other that they are almost sitting on each other's laps. This feels like one of the biggest differences to teaching in men's prisons. Although the men live on the same landing together, they don't know each other on an intimate level. I have to help them become a group. But the women are already a group. They get to decide whether I'm allowed in or not.

A young woman called Imani is sat hunched and clutching a handkerchief. There are empty seats on both sides of her. Opposite Imani is a woman around the same age called Anjela. She is sat with a friend on either side of her, both of them resting their head on her shoulders.

Anjela hums the tune to Rihanna's 'Umbrella'. Her two friends hum along. Imani sniffles.

I try to meet Imani's eye to see if she is OK, but she keeps her gaze fixed on her handkerchief.

I start the class again. I ask them, 'If you lost your memory, would you still be the same person?' A few minutes into the conversation Anjela says, 'I've got a question, Andy. What if you used to be really beautiful, but now you're ugly? You wouldn't be the same person then, would you? Nobody would want you any more.'

Imani bursts into tears, gets up and walks out of the room.

'What's wrong with her?' Anjela says, a smile creeping across her face. 'I didn't do anything.'

While the architecture here is less claustrophobic than the men's prison, it is incredibly socially intense. The conversation hums with a subtext that has existed long before I arrived. Even though I'm the teacher, I'm sometimes the last one in the room to understand what is going on in the discussion.

Halfway through the lesson, an orderly comes in with some tea and biscuits. We take a break. The tea in prison tastes mouldy and bitter. After I drink it, I always suck my teeth to try and get rid of the chemical aftertaste. The women go over to the corner of the room to get their tea and hang out there and chat. I stay at my desk and look over my teaching notes.

Agnes comes over. 'Let me get you a tea,' she says.

Tea is a loophole in the don't-accept-things-from-prisoners rule.

'Thank you,' I say.

Agnes looks pleased. She turns and walks towards the corner of the room. A few seconds later, Sofia comes over to me and puts a small polystyrene cup of tea on my desk.

'You should eat less sugar. You're always yawning,' she says.

I pick up the cup and hold it up to her. 'I alread—'

'What did you have for breakfast?' she asks.

'Toast with butter.'

'You have to eat fruit in the morning.'

Agnes comes over holding a small polystyrene cup. 'Ah.' She turns to Sofia. 'I was getting him tea.'

'I've already got him one,' Sofia says.

We all talk about it and decide that this week I will drink Agnes's tea and next week Sofia will get me tea.

Twenty minutes later, the lesson is back underway. Imani has returned to her seat at the encouragement of two other women who went to comfort her. We continue discussing questions of memory.

'It doesn't matter how old and forgetful your mind gets,' Agnes says, 'you never forget the people you love, do you? That's the most important thing.'

'It's not that you forget people,' Sofia says, 'it's that you remember them wrong, but without realizing that you're remembering them wrong.'

'Well, I don't,' Agnes says.

A few minutes later, I say, 'Neuroscientists say our memory isn't like a video camera. Instead, it reframes and edits events to create a story to fit our current situation. Our memories are always adapting so that we can adapt to whatever is happening now.'

'What are you saying?' Agnes says, her voice trembling. 'I don't have a photo of my father in here with me. My cousin has one of the only photos left of him. When I get out, I'm going to visit her so I can see it. But while I'm waiting for that, every night before I sleep, I make sure I picture my dad's face and hold it there in my mind.'

'I'm sorry. I didn't mean t—'

'Are you saying I'll have spent years remembering him wrong?'

I open my mouth, but I don't know what to say without upsetting Agnes more.

Sofia leans forward in her chair and touches Agnes on the knee. 'Don't torture yourself, my dear. You have to keep your head in jail.'

'I don't want to,' Agnes says.

The following morning, I slice an apple into a bowl and eat it. I realize that prison seems more brutal to me now that I've been inside one containing women. I've heard plenty of men inside say things like, 'Keep your head in jail,' or, 'The sooner you forget about the world outside, the quicker you can do your time.' A lot of them already learnt how to cut themselves off before they stepped through the prison gates. But someone like Agnes isn't native to detachment. Through her, I see afresh how painful the separation of prison is.

Despite the pink paint on the walls, the women's jail ultimately reminds me that prisons are one of the most forceful demonstrations of patriarchal power that there is. I'm used to seeing how the institution pushes men to walk with their shoulders squared and keep their fists half-clenched, always poised for violence. I see that walk in the women's jail too, but I also see how prison pushes some women towards a much more vulnerable and girlish version of themselves. When you enter into the building, you can become an Alsatian or a kitten.

★

Like Agnes, I do not have a photograph of my dad. Ten years ago, a family member showed me one of theirs. For the next two weeks, I had vague feelings of guilt and executioner-type thoughts. I haven't looked at a photo of him since. But I still see men who I momentarily think might be him on the bus, at the urinals in a pub toilet or in a mugshot in the newspaper. I would like to forget my dad, but my imagination won't let me. But that's what shame is – the inability to forget. It's memory at its most insistent.

When Sofia told Agnes to keep her head in jail, she was telling her that she needed to stay in the present. For me, living in the present would mean something like allowing myself out of jail; walking away from my inherited guilt.

Truth

> But behind our lies I am dropping Ariadne's golden thread – for the greatest of all joys is to be able to retrace one's lies, to return to the source and sleep one night a year washed of all superstructures.
>
> ANAÏS NIN

I say to the men, 'The philosopher Sam Harris says that telling a lie is a missed opportunity for deepening our connection with someone else. That includes white lies. He thinks we lie most of the time from weakness. Perhaps the truth is too shameful to admit, or we don't like conflict, so we lie instead. Harris thinks these lies chip away at our relationships. If you lie to someone, it creates a gap in the relationship. Lying can also be stressful and alienating for the person doing the lying. So Harris's philosophy is that we should almost always tell the truth.'

Terry, a man with silver hair and a ruddy complexion, folds his arms. 'What if Sam Harris was approached by a geezer wanting to know the whereabouts of his family. What if Sam Harris notices the geezer looks rather displeased? What does Sam Harris say then?'

I say, 'Harris says those extreme types of situations should have no bearing on our general rule about lying. He makes an analogy to astronauts. When astronauts are in space, they have to take a pill to make sure they don't lose their bone density in the zero gravity. But when astronauts return to earth, there's no need for them to keep taking the pill.'

'Why the fuck is he talking about astronauts?' Terry says.

'He's saying that on extreme occasions, people blackmail or threaten you and you have no choice but to lie, but that doesn't happen most days. So most days, you should still stick to your general rule to be honest.'

'What if someone wanted to rape his sister? Is Sam Harris gonna tell them where she is?' Terry says.

'No. But it's the astronaut thing again. Most of our moral choices take place within a normal atmosphere. Someone telling you they're gonna rape your sister would count as outside of the normal atmosphere. So even if you have to lie when a rapist is looking for your sister, it doesn't mean lying is a good thing to do the other days of the week.'

'OK, what if they were gonna rape his mum?'

'Again, astronauts, Terry,' I say.

'Well, Sam Harris sounds like a very honest man.' An exaggerated smile stretches tightly across his face.

'What's your thought, Terry?' I say.

'I think,' he says, unfolding his arms, 'I think I'm going to take a shit.'

He plants his hand on his knee, groans as he lifts himself off his chair and makes his way to the door.

I was seven. It was coming up to Christmas. I hadn't seen my brother in a couple of months. Mum had told me Jason was away working in a factory and that he would come home once his job had finished in a few months.

On Christmas Eve, I was sitting next to Mum in the front of the car. We were going to visit my brother. We came off the motorway, went down country roads and eventually we arrived at a car park. There was a large sign that said, 'Her Majesty's Prison'.

Confused, I looked at Mum.

'Jason is away at work,' she said. 'He'll be home soon, don't worry. We will only see him for an hour today. Let's have a nice time, OK?'

We got out of the car and went into the building. We stepped into security. Mum gave me a big smile and it made it feel like it would have been wrong to say, 'But this is a prison.' She was allowed to take a packet of four unopened Mars bars in with her. We put my toys, Mum's money, keys and everything else in a locker. Then an officer led us towards the visitors' hall.

Twenty minutes later, I was sitting with Mum in a room with lots of tables with big spaces between them. The windows had bars. We were opposite an empty plastic chair. At the next table there was also a mother and child on one side and an empty chair opposite. A line of men filed through the door wearing bright yellow bibs like you wear at football practice to show what team you're on. One of them was Jason. I was so excited to see him.

He walked over and gave me a hug, his stubble scratching my forehead. An officer told us, 'No touching.'

Jason sat down opposite us. 'Mum probably told you. I'm just busy here doing a bit of work,' he said.

I sat on my hands and kicked one leg back and forth.

Jason sat down. Mum handed Jason a Mars bar. He tore open the packet and took a bite. They talked together in hushed voices. She wanted to know if he was staying out of trouble. I remember that he made a small O shape with his thumb and first finger to show her how tiny the tomatoes served in his meals were. Security guards were patrolling the room. Jason took another bite of the Mars bar and as he pulled it away from his mouth, a string of caramel stretched and broke off, sticking to his chin.

'Do you have a cell to yourself?' Mum whispered.
'They've changed my cell three times already,' Jason said.
'You're in prison,' I said.
They both looked at me.
'I'm just doing a bit of work, Bruv.'
'I've seen *Birds of a Feather*. This is prison.'
Birds of a Feather was a TV show about two women who visited their husbands in jail.
Mum and Jason both cried with laughter.
'This is a prison,' I said.

In January, I went back to school. I sat in my place, opened my workbook and picked up a pencil. A feeling of emptiness came over me. My brother was in prison; how could any of this matter? My teacher told me to write the date at the top of the page. I looked at him and snapped the tip of my pencil against the edge of the table.

I didn't tell anyone that my brother was in prison. I wanted to scream out loud, 'None of this is real. Stop pretending it is.' Once, my teacher was explaining something to us, moving his hands animatedly. I laughed at him. He pulled a serious face, pointed his finger at me and said, 'Is something funny?' Mimicking him, I pulled a serious face, pointed at him and said, 'Is something funny?' He told me to get out of the class. I shrugged and left the room.

My reality had come apart. I was either argumentative or despondent in class. At secondary school, on the rare occasion I did any work, I'd get E and F grades, which I took as confirmation that teachers truly didn't understand anything. Not surprisingly, I left school having failed all but two subjects.

A few months later, some friends of mine were going to the local college open day. I thought there was little point in me joining them since I didn't have the grades. A few months previously, just before my exams, a teacher had photocopied an ex-student's coursework and given it to me to submit under my name. His gesture made me feel like there were teachers who understood that my reality wasn't the same as the one school expected me to live in. So I went to the college and dropped in on a taster philosophy class.

The teacher, Robert, posed the question, 'How do we know this is not just a dream? How do we know any of this is real?'

It was such a relief to hear him ask that question.

Robert allowed me to take the course, even though I didn't have the grades usually required. I found the lessons incredibly exciting.

That was the period of my life when the executioner in my head was at its most condemning. My thoughts were punishingly dichotomous: either I was good or I was bad. I could not live in between those poles. The executioner told me that being in between meant I was on the way to being bad. He stopped the conversation before I could have a second or third thought about who I might be.

But in Robert's classroom, we read about ideas from

philosophers from across the centuries, and in the pages of those books I saw there were people who understood how complex life was. Philosophers seemed to dwell in a place beyond severe either/ors, where nuance was the norm, conversation could carry on and the mind could stretch out. I thought that if I kept doing philosophy I could become uncondemned.

For the first month of the course, I worked hard. But found it difficult. I scored 3/11 on my first essay and 6/18 on my second. Robert wrote in the margin, 'I have to reread a lot of your sentences. Your thoughts don't always make sense.' 'You don't know the half of it,' I wanted to say to him.

I kept working hard, but Robert found my third essay as incomprehensible as the other two. I knew what I was saying, but nobody else did. I assumed my inner world must be inexpressibly particular and I felt hopelessly alienated. Robert asked me to come to his room at lunchtime and he showed me how to write a sentence so that people other than myself could understand my writing. We did this a number of times. But when he was explaining things to me, I was afraid I was going to interrupt and say something cruel to him. I didn't know what the cruel words would be, but I worried it was about to come out of my mouth at any moment. The executioner was uneasy with Robert's kindness.

Robert kept giving me extra support and my grades steadily improved. I went from feeling like I was incomprehensible to knowing the satisfaction of being understood. I'm so grateful to Robert for believing in me during a time when I couldn't easily see good in myself. When I finished studying philosophy, I still had the condemning voice in my head. But now I also had access to a second headspace, one of imagination and possibility. It was like I had obtained a mental version of dual nationality. In the morning I woke up with the executioner in my head. I couldn't banish him from there entirely, but I could cross a bridge to a different island in my mind and enjoy being somewhere else.

I once had a former cage fighter in my class in prison called Dris. He was incredibly muscular, but always stood a little stooped. The crimes for which he'd been convicted could have made him very rich, but in his cell, he scratched the words 'I must not be so greedy' on the wall beside his bed. He was halfway through his second fifteen-year sentence. He saw men arrive and depart. Even the ones in for a few years came and went like extras in a movie. He became too weary to make small talk with anyone new on the wing. It was as though Dris was living in a building with 1,300 bodies with greyed-out faces. But he liked philosophy. It was the only time I saw him look at people rather than over the top of their heads. Once, at the end of a class, he passed me a small slip of paper before he left. It read 'Two-hour holiday. Thank you.' A two-hour holiday was usually what he called a visit from family or friends. In philosophy, Dris got to go somewhere else.

This morning, I arrive at the prison gates but all the staff lockers to stash away my phone are taken. I step inside the creaky Portakabin of the visitor centre. Warm air from the electric heaters makes condensation on the windows. I open one of the lockers and put my phone inside. There is a Prisoners' Families Helpline poster on the wall. It has an image of a young boy with sad eyes next to some text that says, 'Is Daddy working away again?'

I turn the key on my locker and head to teach my class.

A few minutes later, I pass security and step into a room with eight locked cabinets on the walls; each cabinet has a reinforced Perspex front. Inside are rows of keys. I put the pad of my finger on a panel next to the cabinet. The machine verifies my fingerprint and the door of the cabinet opens to me. I take a set of keys and hook them to my belt. I travel through the prison, using my keys to open doors and then lock them behind me. Throughout the morning, I go from the landings to the yard to healthcare to the kitchen to the governor's office and to the segregation unit. When I think back to that Christmas Eve when I was supposed to not know I was in a prison, it almost feels illicit to have these keys on my belt. I keep imagining that an officer is going to approach me and take them off me.

Half an hour later, in my classroom, a new student called Eddie joins the group. Someone talks about how Brazil was the last country to abolish slavery and Eddie interjects to tell everyone he used to have an apartment in Rio overlooking Ipanema beach. Fifteen minutes later, Kosovo is mentioned and Eddie tells us he won a medal fighting there.

Half an hour later, someone disses the Spanish football team and Eddie tells us he once had a holiday romance with a woman who went on to become Miss Spain.

The following week, it is the day before a royal wedding and a student brings to class a packet of chocolate digestive biscuits to share in celebration. Eddie bites into one and says, 'Years ago I got invited to Princess Margaret's house.' As he talks, I see the mush of biscuit on his tongue. 'But I decided not to go in the end.'

Later in the same class, Eddie tells us he once had six numbers come up on the national lottery, but he lost his ticket whilst on a bender with two famous rappers.

The week after, Eddie tells us he has previously shared a cell with some of Britain's most notorious criminals, including Charles Bronson and Abu Hamza. 'Charles Bronson,' he says, 'is one of the nicest blokes you'll ever talk to.'

The next week, Eddie says, 'So I sang a song I wrote at open mic night. And now Ed Sheeran is making a killing off it.'

When Eddie first interrupted people with these stories, the other men would give him a heavy look. Now they stare into space. Nobody bothers to ask him to sing an Ed Sheeran tune or what Miss Spain's hair smells like.

Eddie has been in the class for about two months when I write on the board 'Truth = Goodness?'

I say, 'Plato argued that the philosopher kings would be ideal leaders of the state. A philosopher king is someone with a masterful grasp of geometry and mathematics. Plato thought that because the philosopher kings understood abstract truths, they would also understand what was good. Truth equals goodness. So, these philosopher kings would be the best rulers.'

'What, like having Stephen Hawking at Downing Street?' a student says.

'Kind of,' I say. 'In fact, there is something like a real-world example. When Israel was first formed, Albert Einstein was invited to be the president, but he declined.'

'No he wasn't,' says Eddie.

'He was,' I say.

'Wouldn't happen.'

I scratch my head. 'I've read about it.'

Eddie wags his finger. 'I spent a lot of time in Israel when I was a consultant. Einstein – never.'

I smile to try to hide the fact my nostrils are flaring with irritation. I look to the other students and point to 'Truth = Goodness?' on the board. 'Do you agree?' I say.

A few hours later, I arrive home, switch on my laptop and search 'Einstein declined Israel presidency'. I find an article that confirms Einstein was, in fact, offered the opportunity to be the president of Israel. At the top of the page, it has the iconic black-and-white photo of Einstein pulling a face. His narrow, pointed tongue appears from below his grey moustache.

I print off the article and put it in my teaching folder.

A few days later, in the women's prison, the students are trickling into the class. A woman called Stacey sits at a table in the corner and adds a few extra lines to a letter she is writing. She wears a grey hoodie with the sleeves pushed up to the elbows. She has a tattoo of her daughter's name on her inner forearm. I ask her how she is. She finishes the sentence she is writing, her tongue pressed against her top teeth, and says, 'I have to write to my girlfriend every day. She didn't believe the letters were from me at first. Outside my handwriting is always so scruffy, but I've got time in here. My handwriting has become so neat.'

The rest of the women arrive. Stacey joins the circle. To my right is a nineteen-year-old called Britney. She wears dark purple lipstick and has a missing tooth in the corner of her smile. Opposite her is Leanne, a Glaswegian woman in her late twenties. She is talking to her neighbour about a mental health advice leaflet that the prison gave out earlier this week. It recommends regular exercise and meditation. Leanne is upset that the leaflets also said to 'Spend time with people you enjoy being with.'

'Honestly,' Leanne says. 'It can't take much to get a job in this place. You don't even have to live in the real world.'

I feel slightly self-conscious. I expect Leanne thinks of me as another one who doesn't live in the real world.

A few minutes later, the class gets underway. I say, 'In 1944, a Japanese soldier called Hiroo Onoda was sent to fight on an island in the Philippines. Before his commanding officer Major Taniguchi left, he told Onoda he'd return for him, and Onoda was forbidden to surrender.'

Leanne is scribbling over a magazine on her lap, filling with black biro the whites of the eyes and teeth of a model in a skincare advert.

'The following year, the Allies took the island. Onoda hid in the jungle. He survived on bananas, coconuts, and raided local farms when he could. Half a year later, he came across a leaflet in the jungle telling him that the war had ended months ago. He believed the leaflet was a fake, that it was the enemy trying to trick them into surrender.'

Britney guffaws. Leanne looks irritated with her.

I say, 'At the end of 1945, the locals got a plane, flew over the jungle and dropped leaflets with General Yamashita's letter of surrender on it. Onoda didn't believe the letter. He thought that there was no way Japan could have lost the war and that this was the Allies trying to trick him again.'

I try to project my voice a little more to see if I can get

Leanne's attention. 'More leaflets were dropped, newspapers from Japan, photos and letters from the soldiers' loved ones.'

Leanne keeps scribbling, her head down.

'Onoda didn't believe any of it. Japanese delegates were sent. They walked through the jungle shouting through a megaphone. Onoda thought this was probably Japanese soldiers who had been caught by the enemy and forced to trick him into surrender.'

'He has to be paranoid,' Stacey says.

'Onoda had been in the jungle for thirty years when a Japanese student travelling in the Philippines found him. The student tells him the war is over, but Onoda says that he will not believe that the war is over unless his commanding officers return to tell him so.'

I ask the class, 'Should Onoda believe the war has ended?'

'Of course he should,' says Britney.

'Why?' Leanne asks.

'Because it's the truth.'

'Truth is just a word,' Leanne says. 'My lawyer told me to wear a long-sleeve shirt for my trial to hide my tattoos. What difference does that make to whether I'm innocent or guilty if I have tattoos on my arm?'

'But you know if you're innocent or guilty. The truth is real to you,' Britney says.

Leanne, scribbling on the magazine, says, 'The truth is real, but it doesn't really matter.'

The teeth of the blonde model in her magazine were now two-thirds black.

'Surely the truth matters if Onoda is gonna live in reality,' I say.

'The world has forgotten about him,' Leanne says. 'His

family and kids have probably moved on. He thinks he's fighting the Americans and now there's probably a McDonald's in his hometown. Nobody will remember him. He won't recognize anything.' Still looking down and scribbling, 'Can't he just believe what he wants?'

'But don't they say the truth will set you free?' Britney says.

'Oh please,' says Leanne. 'Andy, does he leave the jungle or not?'

'The student goes back to Japan and finds Major Taniguchi working in a bookshop. He tells him about the situation and Taniguchi travels to the island. When Taniguchi gets there, he finds that Onoda is wearing the same clothes as when he gave him the order to not surrender three decades ago. His uniform is in immaculate condition.'

Leanne stops her pen and lifts her head to look at me. Her eyes look bright with pain.

'His rifle is also impeccably kept. Taniguchi has a choice,' I say. I feel Leanne's eyes burning into me. My voice wavers slightly. 'He can either tell Onoda that the war has ended, or he can tell Onoda to keep holding his position.'

I say, 'What should Taniguchi tell Onoda?'

Stacey leans forward in her chair and says, 'It's dangerous to tell him. It could be like waking up a sleepwalker.'

'He can't sleep forever,' Britney says.

'If it was only five years after the war was over, but this is thirty years!' Stacey says.

'Five years or thirty years – it don't change the truth,' Britney says.

Stacey says, 'I did six years once. When I came out, everything felt like it was happening so fast. Time in here is different, everything is slow and as soon as I was let out of the gates, it was like I had to run just to keep up with everyone else. Just doing the basics almost killed me and that was only after six years. Onoda might never catch up.'

'I still believe he can adapt,' Britney says.

Leanne scoffs.

'And it's dishonest if he doesn't tell him,' Britney says.

'At my trial, they said they would decide if I had lied or not by whether a normal person would find me honest,' Leanne says. 'What does that mean – a normal person who is a judge, a normal prisoner, a normal soldier living in the jungle for thirty years? Tell me what a normal person is.'

'Doesn't Onoda deserve honesty?' I say.

'Does Taniguchi tell him the truth?' Leanne says.

'Yes,' I say.

'Well, how does the story end?' Leanne says.

'Taniguchi tells Onoda that the war is over. Onoda pulls back the bolt of his rifle and unloads the bullets. He lays his gun down. He says everything went black. He wishes that he had died with his men in battle thirty years ago. He could no longer understand what his last thirty years as a soldier had been for.'

Leanne puts her pen back on the page and continues shading over the model's face.

An hour later, the class ends. I leave the prison and go into the visitor centre. On the wall, I see a poster advertising a helpline. It has a picture of a little girl and the words 'I miss Mummy'. I unlock my locker, take out my phone and wallet and leave.

★

A few days later, in the men's prison, Eddie doesn't attend philosophy because he's meeting his caseworker. I want to give him this week's reading about Descartes and I also want to show him the article that confirms Einstein was offered the Israeli presidency. I head down the landing. Everything is grey. Everyone is yawning. The air is filled with the smells of unwashed men and the sound of daytime TV. I get to Eddie's cell and the door is still open. I stand just outside his doorway. He has placed an opened carton of UHT milk on the frame of his open window to help it stay cool. Eddie's lying on his mattress, staring at the ceiling. Next to his bed is a toilet roll that's down to the last few sheets.

'I've got two things for you,' I say.

Eddie gets to his feet and steps towards me. I pull out the Descartes reading from my file and give it to him. He peeks his head out of the cell, looking left then right and then takes a step back. He bites the nail of his thumb.

I flick through my folder and half pull out the Einstein article when Eddie says, 'Two blokes took my telly. They walked in here and flicked through the channels and I said, "What the fuck you doing," and they both just laughed. They unplugged it and took off with it.'

I look in his cell. A fine dust covers the table but for a clean square where the TV was.

He says, 'They just left and I couldn't do anything. I'm out of here in seven months if I stay on good behaviour, but those two are doing ten years, they can play by their own rules. They know they can take the piss and there's nothing I can do back.'

'I'm sorry, Eddie,' I say.

'I'm a black belt in karate as well.'

'Have you told security?'

Eddie darts his eyes to the side. He doesn't want to be a grass.

'But you'll see those men every day. What if they keep doing it?' I say.

Eddie steps away, lies down on his bed and groans, 'What's the other thing you wanted?'

I look at the article half hanging out of my folder. I can see the image of Einstein sticking his tongue out.

'Sorry, Eddie,' I say.

He lifts his head off the pillow to look at me.

'There wasn't another thing,' I say.

Eddie drops his head back onto the pillow. I tuck the article back into my folder.

Looking

> The gaze is a singular act: to look at something
> is to fill your whole life with it.
>
> OCEAN VUONG

Forty years after leaving Auschwitz, Primo Levi published an essay called *Shame*, in which he went to a friend for help in making sense of why it was that he had survived the Lager when others had not. His friend told him he had lived so he could 'bear witness' to what the others went through.

Twenty-five years ago, when Mum and I were visiting Jason in prison, our time ran out and the officers took him back to his cell. Mum and I went through the exit and stepped outside into the car park. I felt there was something wrong that I was getting to leave and Jason wasn't. Mum and I got in the car and pulled away. I turned around, knelt on the seat and stared out the back window at the prison. Mum told me to sit down and face the front, but I couldn't look away.

This morning, I'm walking down the landing and I hear a scream behind me. I turn around and see a man who doesn't look much older than twenty being escorted by six officers. They're holding him by the arms. He struggles to break free and his long black hair falls across one of their faces.

'He was wanking at me,' the man shouts.

He has a bloodied cheekbone and the V-neck of his white T-shirt is torn. There is wild rage in his eyes.

'Wanking in my fucking face!'

The officers carry him down the landing towards the segregation unit to calm him down.

An officer called Fowler tells me that Jonesy – the man escorted to the seg – had a new cellmate move in last night. This morning, Jonesy woke up to his cellmate masturbating in his face. Jonesy jumped out of bed and pushed him against the wall. The other man fought back, his erection poking out. Security had to break them up.

'Oh my god,' I say.

Fowler laughs nervously. A few men on the landing are jeering at Jonesy and making a wanking gesture with their hands. An officer shouts, 'Free flow.' Fowler leaves to assume his position.

I stand and watch the officers carrying Jonesy down the stairs to the seg.

Levi tried to bear witness as best he could, but it didn't make him feel any less troubled about the fact he was alive. The very fact that he was able to observe others' suffering reminded him that he had survived while others hadn't. Bearing witness only multiplied his shame.

After I finish work, I'm sat on the train that's waiting on the platform. Each time I blink, I picture the torn neckline of Jonesy's white T-shirt. I clench my jaw.

The train pulls away and the atoms holding reality together come apart. The conductor walks through the carriage but my brain can't put together how he is moving forward just by putting his legs one after the other. He goes through the automatic doors, which open with an exaggerated 'whoosh', like a sound effect on a cheap movie set. The table in front seems far away, as though if I were to put my hand out to touch it, I wouldn't be able to reach. I look out of the window at the city and I struggle to believe the buildings and roads and cars actually exist. There is nothing there behind the glass.

Towards the end of *Shame*, Levi described feeling an anguish so absolute that it was like he was living in a crushed universe where the human spirit had been extinguished. Everything had come apart. A year after publishing the essay, Levi threw himself from the third-floor landing outside his apartment and died on the stairwell.

Two weeks after seeing Jonesy get carried to the seg, I'm on the threes and I hear shouting and banging from below. I look down through the metal anti-suicide nets. On the twos, some officers are carrying a man to the seg.
    I feel light-headed. But I can't look away.

Laughter

> Humour: the divine flash that reveals the
> world in its moral ambiguity and man in his
> profound incompetence to judge others;
> humour: the intoxicating relativity of human
> things; the strange pleasure that comes of
> the certainty that there is no certainty.
>
> MILAN KUNDERA

Jerome walks into my classroom for the first time in over a year. I haven't seen him since he was in my class about luck. He has been released and reconvicted. He has got skinnier and his trembling hand seems to have become more severe, but his goofy smile hasn't changed.

I say, 'The ancient philosopher Chrysippus was at the Olympiad games when a donkey came up to the table and started to eat his figs. Chrysippus shouted, "Now give the donkey a pure wine to wash down the figs!" and burst out laughing. He laughed so hard that he could no longer stand. He fell on the ground, shaking uncontrollably and foaming at the mouth. People tried to help him but they couldn't and he died.'

'That's such a beautiful way to go. Like dying from sex,' says Jerome.

'Wouldn't it be better if he was laughing at someone else's joke?' I say.

'Then it would be murder. The Old Bill would be all over it, especially with the foaming at the mouth part.'

'It's not embarrassing that it was his own joke?' I ask.

'He's dead. Isn't it enough to be embarrassed when you're alive?' Jerome says.

On Saturday afternoon, at my nan's house, Mum passes me her phone. She steps back and puts her arm around Uncle Frank. I hold up the phone and try to get a picture of them that won't be upstaged by the large oval-framed picture of Rhett Butler from *Gone with the Wind*. I count down 'three-two-one' and Frank pushes out his top row of false teeth with his tongue. I press the button.

I show Mum the photo. Frank appears to have the world's most pronounced overbite. Behind his head there's the swirl pattern of the textured wall paint. We all laugh at the photo except for Nan, who sits on the sofa, looking into the distance instead of watching the Sunday morning cooking programme she has on at blaring volume.

'Do you want a cup of tea, Nan?' I say.

'I feel so rotten, putting him in there,' Nan says.

She's looking at the urn with Grandad's ashes on the fireplace. My grandad worked as a gravedigger for over a decade. So did his brothers and some of his children.

'But Grandad asked to be cremated,' I say.

'I just feel horrible, knowing I put him through that fire,' she says.

'He made an informed choice, Nan,' I say.

Twenty minutes later, Nan goes to the bathroom and I turn the TV volume down seven notches. Frank sits on the arm of the sofa, takes out a pouch of tobacco and a cigarette paper. He's in a good mood, telling me and Mum stories.

'I was doing six months, but I'd also been nicked for

thieving something else and that was gonna get me another three months,' he says.

The corners of Mum's mouth point into a grin. I'm also poised to laugh.

'I knew I was gonna get guilty, and my solicitor said they would probably give it to me consecutive rather than concurrent. On the morning, the screws got me out of my cell and took me to court. I only went for the change of scenery. At the court, I've gone to the toilet and my co-d Charlie has come in a few minutes later. He takes out this spliff from his pocket and we have a puff in a cubicle. Only thing is, it's made us piss ourselves laughing. The screw knocks on the door, telling us that we're about to begin, but we're laughing and laughing. Charlie throws the spliff down the toilet and the screws walk us into the courthouse. Charlie's snorting. I'm biting into my fist. I'm stood before the judge covering my face with my hands.'

Me and Mum are giggling. Frank sprinkles tobacco on the Rizla, licks the edge of the paper and closes the cigarette.

'The hearing took five minutes,' he says. 'I spent all of that hunched over the table, convulsing with laughter. The judge gave us both Guilty and then he has to sentence us. I've lifted my head off the table. I'm bright fucking red by this stage. The judge said, "Your crime was appalling" and all that bollocks – and then he's gone, "but I can see you're crying. You're beginning to recognize the error of your ways." Then he goes and gives us the sentence concurrently. That sets me off laughing all over again.'

A few minutes later, I'm with my uncle in the kitchen. We're waiting for the kettle to boil. He rolls a cigarette and tells me about a trip he took to the coast a decade ago. The tide was going out. He went into the sea up to his knees and stood there quietly. Seals swam around him. They stared at him from a few metres away.

'We should go there,' I say.

'Yes. Let's wait for a clear day, so we can see everything properly,' he says.

Since Frank got out of prison, he and I have talked about the many things we will go to see at the coast once we get a clear day. But many clear days have come and gone without Frank and me leaving the sofa. Yet we still continue to talk about the birds, seals and sky we will one day go and see together. It is as if the clear day is part of our alternate future rather than our real one.

The kettle boils. Frank makes tea and hands me one. He tucks his roll-up behind his ear and we go back into the living room and sit down.

Over the afternoon, there's a constant babble of laughter in the living room as Frank tells me and Mum stories. My laughter makes him laugh, which makes Mum laugh, which makes me laugh, which makes Frank laugh again. The wall that separates me from my uncle becomes more permeable as we pass laughter back and forth to each other.

At about five o'clock, Frank taps his roll-up on his knee. He tells us a story from when he was in Canterbury prison thirty years ago and fighting with a gang from Essex. I listen with a grin fixed to my face.

'The screws have gone round locking up everyone, except for our cell. So, I've filled the kettle with water and boiled it. Then I've just waited. A minute and I've boiled it again. Me and Vinnie are watching the door. I just keep boiling the kettle. There's all fucking steam in the air. Then we hear footsteps. I pick up the kettle and open the lid and three geezers from the Essex mob have stormed in.'

Frank looks admiringly into the distance.

'I threw water right in the bloke's face,' Frank says.

I lose my grin. I'm sober with shock and disgust.

'You should have seen the geezer's face,' Frank says. He puts his hands on the sides of his face and stretches his skin, his eyes and lips curling downwards. He sticks his tongue out and moans, 'Whuuuur!'

I fold over laughing. Mum has to hold her stomach because she's laughing so hard. Frank looks delighted with himself.

I put a hand over my mouth to try and stop. I take a deep breath, take my hand away and try to calm down, but tears are running down Mum's face and Frank is laughing at her and that sets me off again.

A few hours later, I'm walking home. The sky is clear but for a few clouds that are as fine as vapour. At home, I put a teabag in a mug and boil the kettle. I pour in the hot liquid. The water turns dark.

I stir the tea with a spoon and the steam brushes the backs of my fingers. I put the spoon down and rest the pad of my finger on the surface of the tea. It doesn't feel hot, but then my hand whips back. My fingertip is sore. It's turning red. I dig my thumb into it to get a more intimate definition of the pain.

I turn on the cold tap and put my finger under the water until it goes numb.

★

The next morning, I still feel a tenderness in my finger as I write with my whiteboard pen. Several men sit around the table. Jerome boasts about how his football team won yesterday. He banged his cell door each time they scored during the highlights on *Match of the Day* last night. Dev, a gangly man in his forties, keeps yawning today. I ask him if he's OK, but he folds his arms on the table and lays his head in the crease of his elbow, using his bicep as a pillow.

A man called Alistair walks in, sits down and slouches nonchalantly in his chair. He wears a pair of delicate rimless glasses and he's the first prisoner I've seen wearing slip-on shoes.

I close the door and get the class underway. I say, 'The surrealist artist André Breton tells a story about a man led to the gallows. He is to be hanged. The noose is tied around his neck. The executioner asks if he has any last words. The man turns to the executioner and says, "Are you sure this is safe?"'

'Ha. Excellent,' Alistair says.

I ask, 'Is there anything better the man could have said?'

'It doesn't matter what he says,' Dev says, his words muffled by the table.

Alistair says, 'Well of course he could have recited the complete works of Shakespeare. Or the complete works of Christopher Marlowe, although Marlowe didn't write quite as much as Shakespeare. But either would have bought him a bit more life.'

'He could have said sorry. Asked for forgiveness,' Ian says.

Ian has dry and cracked skin. A T-shirt swamps his skinny body. He has red scratch marks on his inner forearm and speaks with an angry, mumbly voice.

Alistair says, 'I'm afraid I don't see why he should have to say sorry. Maybe he'd only stolen a loaf of bread. What the state is doing to him is far worse than what he has done.'

'I bet it wasn't a loaf of bread,' Ian says.

Alistair flicks his wrist. 'The time for sorry is before that. This isn't about his crime any more. This is about the end of his life. This is his moment. They are taking his life and that's wrong, thank you very much. If he says sorry, then he is legitimizing his execution and the whole set-up.'

'So, if we say sorry for our crimes, are we saying prison is good, then?' Ian says.

Alistair shrugs. 'The state doesn't care if you're actually sorry. They just want to see you on your knees.'

Ian says, 'Isn't the man a loser? Isn't it pathetic making a joke as you're about to die? People in here tell me my face would break if I smiled. I'm fine with that. I don't want to be some jackass who thinks it's funny to be in prison.'

'It doesn't matter what he says,' Dev groans, his head still on the table. 'It won't change anything.'

We all look at Dev, expecting him to say more, but he keeps his head on the table.

I say, 'Is Dev right? Does it change anything if the man tells a joke before they kill him?'

Ian scratches his forearm. He says, 'The joke changes nothing. But if he said sorry, that might help to take away some of the pain he's caused his victims.'

'I can't see André Breton doing restorative justice,' Alistair scoffs. 'By making the joke, the man stops the executioner from winning. He's letting the executioner know that he can take his life, but he can't take anything else from him.'

'What's wrong with restorative justice?' Ian says.

'For one thing, it has such an inelegant name.' Alistair runs his fingers through his hair and changes the cross of his legs.

A few minutes later, Ian says, 'Have you seen those old Victorian photos where the faces look so sullen? That's because it took the camera half an hour to take the photo and you can't smile for half an hour straight. If someone tells you they see life as a comedy, they're lying.'

Alistair inspects his fingernails.

Dev groans. He lifts his head and rubs his eyes.

'What do you think, Dev?' I ask.

'Last week, my cellmate ordered a little packet of 15p Skittles, but on Friday morning when we got our canteen, the Skittles weren't there. He went quiet. Didn't say anything all weekend. Then last night, at about nine-thirty, he started banging the door, shouting that he wanted his Skittles. When the guvs came, they told him he'd have to wait until next week. He shouted at them, so they closed the viewing hatch and walked away. Then he took the round wire aerial off the TV and put it around his neck. He was threatening to do himself in unless they brought him some Skittles.'

'Dev, that must have been so distressing,' I say.

'Yeah, *Match of the Day* was about to start,' he says.

Jerome throws his head back and laughs.

'I hate you, Dev,' Jerome says. 'Just when I was starting to believe I was turning into a good person, you make me laugh at shit like that.'

Dev drops his head back on the table.

★

A few hours later, I'm walking home and thinking of Alistair's idea about how the condemned man jokes to stop the executioner from winning. One of the most oppressive things about the executioner in my head is how it removes my access to humour or playfulness. It makes my every action desperate – when I meet the eye of a stranger on the train, when I try to fall asleep and when I walk up to the top of the hill near my house, I'm hoping for forgiveness. When my grandfather had dementia and he was dying in hospital he kept saying to the nurses, 'Is there something I should be doing now? Should I have done something?' He was raised in an orphanage that was strict about teaching the children duty and obedience. That stayed with him when the rest of his personality had fallen away. I worry that when I'm dying I'll keep saying to the nurses, 'Have I done something bad? I'm not going to do something bad, am I?' That's why I admire the man at the gallows when he says 'Are you sure this is safe?' His irony isn't only to defend himself against condemnation; it's also intended to undermine the possibility of his redemption. He escapes the guilt-forgiveness bind which the executioner put him in. He jokes so that he can die on his own terms.

On the day my brother told me about how he got the scar on his thigh, he also told me how, about five years before, some drug dealers informed Jason and his mate Tobias that they would be repaying their debts by running six kilos of cocaine across town. Tobias said he didn't want to. The dealers put him in a car with a very wound-up Rottweiler and locked all the doors. Tobias crossed his arms over his face to try to protect himself. The dealers watched on and laughed. Jason laughed too.

'You laughed?' I said.

'If I didn't laugh, I was next,' he said.

The day after my class on Breton, I'm in the women's prison. Anjela and her friend Britney ask me when the philosophy course will end. I tell them we have three weeks left.

'Oh no!' Anjela says.

'Are you sure?' says Britney.

'I'm afraid the class has to end sometime,' I say, feeling proud about how much these two enjoy my teaching.

Britney and Anjela squeeze each other tight.

Anjela says to me, 'We're on different wings. We only come here to see each other.'

'Oh,' I say.

'Is it really just three weeks?' Britney asks.

Thirty minutes later, I ask all the women in the class to swap places and share their thoughts with someone they don't normally talk with to help pollinate more ideas. Britney and Anjela react to this request by clutching their arms around one another. They stay put, Britney resting her head on Anjela's shoulder. A few minutes later, small groups of women are debating the philosophy of time. Britney and Anjela face each other and sing 'Pat-a-cake, pat-a-cake, bake-me-a-cake,' clapping their hands against each other's. The two shriek with laughter because Anjela has accidentally slapped Britney on her boob.

On Thursday night, I'm preparing a class on Nietzsche and laughter. Nietzsche believes life is a very serious matter. There's no God, the universe is tragically indifferent to us and we will die alone. However, Nietzsche sees this as no reason to adopt a spirit of gravity and po-faced solemnity. Seriousness is the very reason to laugh. When you realize that the brutal emptiness of existence is itself the ultimate joke, you laugh a laugh that raises you above the abyss. There's no reality too gruesome that this 'laughter from the height' cannot overcome. The higher the seriousness, the more elevating the laughter.

I think of my uncle Frank. There is not much in life that is too tragic for him not to joke about. I admire how he can laugh himself above pain. Yet it is the fact he is above pain that puts a distance between us.

On Friday morning, I tell the women a story from Nietzsche about the laughter that overcomes tragedy.

I say, 'A character called Zarathustra finds a young shepherd writhing around on the side of the road. A heavy black snake hangs out of his mouth. Zarathustra tries to pull the snake off the shepherd, but he can't because the snake has attached itself to the shepherd's throat with its teeth.'

Britney and Anjela put their hands over their mouths and wheeze with laughter.

I carry on. 'The shepherd sinks his teeth into the snake's flesh. He bites all the way through the body. The tail drops to the floor. The shepherd gets to his feet, spits out the snake's head and breaks into a terrifying, radiant laughter. Zarathustra is awestruck. He has never heard a laugh like it anywhere before.'

'Maybe he still has a bit of snake in his mouth?' Anjela says.

Britney grips on to Anjela's arm so she doesn't fall off her chair.

★

Wittgenstein said that it would be possible to write a legitimate work of philosophy consisting entirely of jokes. My friend Johnny would disagree. He and I were frequently held in detention together at school for piss-taking. At seventeen, when I got into philosophy, he thought I'd taken an overdose of seriousness.

He went on to become a gardener. He has round shoulders, strong arms and is almost always bronzed and cheerful. In my late twenties, I had one of my first pieces of writing published. On his sofa, I opened the piece on my laptop and placed it in front of Johnny. He read the first three or four hundred words, set the laptop aside and got up to make himself a cup of tea.

I followed him into the kitchen. 'Don't you like it?'

'I just thought it'd be funnier,' he said.

'It wasn't supposed to be funny.'

'I know.' He smiled and shrugged. 'I just thought it'd be funnier.'

A few years ago, I wrote a piece with the explicit intention of making the reader laugh. It got accepted for publication, which I took as confirmation that I had succeeded in being funny. I messaged Johnny the link to the piece.

The next day he messaged back.

'Andy, that was heartbreaking.'

When I was seven, I sat on the living room floor of my nan's house with my brother, watching a videotape of *The Krays*, a biopic about the two East End gangsters who were at large in the 1960s. I was in a sulk because he had a mohawk and I wanted one too, but my mum wouldn't let me. On the TV, the Kray twins pinned a man to the wall, held a knife horizontally over his mouth and pressed into his flesh. Blood welled up around the blade. I covered my eyes with my hands. My brother told me that kind of wound was called a Chelsea smile because the scar it left would make it look like the man had a permanent grin.

A few minutes later, Nan came into the room and saw we were watching *The Krays*. 'Nobody mugged old ladies in them days. The Krays'd sort them out if they did,' she said.

She thumbed her thick gold earrings.

Nan said, 'Her from number nineteen was in the pub once and the Krays came in. They bought everyone drinks. They was handsome, you know.'

That night, I lay awake in bed, terrified that someone was about to come into my room and cut a permanent smile into my face; that my nan found the Krays attractive made me afraid that she might be the one to let them into the house.

On Sunday, I arrive at my nan's house. She opens the door and pulls her open cardigan around her body. I give her a hug and I can feel the bones in her back against my arms. We go into the living room. *The Krays* VHS is still on the shelf. The red text on the cover has faded.

Frank is upstairs in his room and has been for the last three days. He occasionally gets depressed, telling us that he doesn't see any point in living any more. His mood becomes more oppressive until he finds it almost impossible to speak. Unable to be the comedian that everyone expects him to be, he shuts himself up in his room.

'Has he been smoking a lot of weed?' I ask Nan.

'I haven't smelt any,' she says.

'That doesn't sound good. Has he been eating?'

'Only bits. It's not that he doesn't want to see you though, Andy,' Nan says.

I go to the bottom of the stairs and look up at his closed bedroom door. I can't hear a television playing or any movement from inside.

'I hope you're OK, Unc. I just wanted to tell you I love you,' I say, through the door.

He doesn't answer

I tap the door.

He doesn't open it.

The next morning, I walk down the landing and I see a cell that has no door, just a thick sheet of Perspex over the door frame. An officer dressed in civilian clothing sits on a swivel chair outside the cell. The man inside has recently attempted suicide and so is now under twenty-four-hour watch. I slow my walk as I pass and glance in. He's lying face down on the mattress.

I walk to my room and on the whiteboard I write, 'Philosophy is a preparation for death – Socrates'. I set the chairs up in a circle. An officer in the corridor shouts, 'Free flow!' I hear the men approaching.

Ian arrives. A two-inch hole has formed in the shoulder of his T-shirt since last week. Alistair, Jerome and the other men file in and sit in the circle.

I say, 'Breton said gallows humour was "the mortal enemy of sentimentality". But is it dangerous to make an enemy of our sentimentality?'

Alistair looks at me over the top of his glasses.

I continue, 'Nietzsche said, "A joke is an epitaph on the death of a feeling." Kierkegaard was another who warned that humour could cost the soul. He says the joker passes on their chance to express themselves sincerely from the heart.'

'Robin Williams. He killed himself,' Ian says.

I ask, 'Should the man in Breton's story have said something more heartfelt?'

'He was coming from the heart,' Alistair says. 'If he'd said, "Are you sure this is safe?" and at the same time, you noticed the crotch area was filling with piss, then he wasn't heartfelt. Or if he'd stayed up all the night before scripting different lines, that wouldn't have been heartfelt. But he surprised himself by saying, "Are you sure this is safe?" It was purely improvised. You can't get more heartfelt than that.'

'That just means he's a good actor,' Ian says.

Alistair sighs. 'You want him to say sorry, but when a man with a noose around his neck says sorry, then I'm afraid it means nothing.'

'You only care about if he carries off the line well. Not if he's being real,' Ian says.

'Look, some jokes cover the truth. Other jokes come from the truth. His joke shows, truthfully, how fucked up his situation is,' Alistair says.

'He's taking the piss so he doesn't have to face the situation like so many morons in this place. You know why prison is always full of piss-takers? Because piss-takers never sort their life out.'

In the classroom, I look at Alistair. He reclines in his chair and listens to Ian with a faint smile resting on his face.

I say, 'The poet Robert Frost said that we joke to avoid the fact that, at bottom, life is not a joke.'

'Bless him,' Alistair says.

'He said that "humour is the most engaging form of cowardice",' I say.

Jerome says, 'Years ago I was at a house party where things got out of hand. Some people had guns and there was a shoot-out. I dropped to the floor and played dead till it was over. A few years later, I was in jail. I told the bloke I was bunking with about it and how I'd played dead. He pissed himself laughing. I asked him what was so funny. He just said, "You're jokes", and kept laughing.'

'He thought you were a coward. But Frost would say he was a coward for laughing,' Ian says.

'He wouldn't have been fucking laughing if he was there,' Jerome says.

Alistair changes the cross of his legs. He waves his hand and says, 'I'm sorry I can't be as pure as Frost. The fact is, a coward would have stood on the gallows and begged for his life. Breton's man was brave. He essentially gave the finger to the executioner, but as deftly as possible. There are more violent ways to rebel, but he decided to make a joke. He chose the most good-natured form of defiance.'

'He was going to die anyway. There were no consequences for whatever he said. That's not really bravery. He was given a free shot,' Ian says.

Alistair takes his glasses off and cleans them using the bottom of his polo shirt. His face looks completely different. He has small bird-like eyes, and the skin beneath looks tough and sinewy.

'It's the sacred versus the profane, that's all. Frost thinks jokes are profane,' Alistair says.

He puts his glasses back on. His eyes look sharp again.

He says, 'He's saying that life isn't a joke because he thinks life is sacred. That's all.'

Twenty minutes later, I exit the prison gates and take my phone out of my locker to find I have a missed call from Mum. I stand in the car park, upwind from a group of smoking prison officers and call her back.

Mum answers. 'It's your uncle Frank.'

'What's happened? Is he OK?' I say.

The officers' smoke drifts into my face. My eyes sting.

'He's had a letter from the benefits office. They want to declare him fit for work,' Mum says.

'I'll be there right away.'

An hour later, in my nan's living room, my uncle paces up and down. I sit cross-legged on the floor at the coffee table, flicking through the thirty-page form. It asks for Frank to list his details, qualifications, criminal record, mental health record and so on.

'How am I supposed to fucking know what to put down? You've got a way with words though, Andy,' Frank says.

Frank goes and smokes on the balcony. It's a relief to see him out of his room. Nan brings me a plate of six Wagon Wheels and two custard slices. I fill out the first pages of the form. I feel excited at the prospect of answering a comprehensive list of questions about my uncle as if his life written in my handwriting could provide proof of our relationship.

Frank has only ever had one job. In his twenties, he worked in a warehouse, which is remarkable given the dozens of warehouses he has burgled. He was there for eighteen months before the manager told him the business had gone bankrupt.

My uncle got a reference but found no other employer willing to take a chance on him. However, 'work' is a common word in Frank's vocabulary. He often describes how Vinnie and he 'work together'. Frank has worked for five decades, all across the country. He worked through the night and on Sundays. He still gets phone calls from people asking him if he wants 'a bit of work'. In arguments with his ex-wife, he'd say, 'I work hard for this family.' But Frank is too old for burgling now. The welfare office is trying to declare him fit for work just as he's retired.

I look back over what I have written in the mental health section of the form. It looks so extreme. I go out onto the balcony. Frank is smoking a roll-up that's right down to the filter.

'I just want to check you're happy with what I've put,' I say.

'Just tell them I'm fucked,' he says.

'I've written this: feelings of hopelessness, withdrawn, short-term memory loss, mood swings.'

'That's blinding, Andy.'

'Panic attacks, thoughts of suicide, feelings of dread.'

'Beautiful.'

Race

> I could never shake the suspicion that everything about me was the consequence of a series of improbable accidents . . . As I saw it, even my strongest feelings and convictions might easily be otherwise, had I been the child of the next family down the hall.
>
> ZADIE SMITH

Yesterday afternoon I arrived at work and at security there was a queue of prisoners' family and friends who had come to visit. I joined the line. In front of me was a boy with his mother. I saw in his face the mixture of excitement and dread which I recognized from when I had visited my brother inside when I was a kid. I smiled at the boy. He squeezed his mother's hand. They both went through security and then I went in after them.

Stepping into prison sometimes feels like I'm walking a path of continuity from my past to my present; from prison visitor to prison teacher, from my family to myself. Going to my grandmother's on a Sunday afternoon and hanging out with my uncle can feel like travelling that path in the opposite direction. The profane, absurd and bathetic conversation often reminds me of being in my classroom.

During my first year in the job, I was renting a room in an ex-council flat on the North Peckham Estate. The local area was known as 'Little Lagos', on account of how many Nigerian people live in the area. Two minutes from my door there were cafes serving jollof rice, plantain and puff puff, but I spent most of my time working on my MacBook in one of the cafes that had recently opened with Peckham's gentrification. One morning, I was halfway through teaching a class in prison when a black man who looked like he was only about nineteen walked into the room. He picked up a pen and wrote a postcode on the board in graffiti-style letters.

'Do you need something?' I asked.

He dropped the pen on the floor and walked out, leaving the door open behind him. The postcode he'd drawn in the board referred to an area his gang was fighting another gang over. It was also two streets from where I lived.

That evening when I got home, I thought about that young man. We both came from working-class backgrounds, but where I went on to university, to become a teacher and to return to an estate as a private renter instead of a council tenant, he went to prison. When I was his age, a philosophy teacher was giving me extra help in his lunch hour.

Throughout my adult life, whenever I've been in polite society and mentioned that my dad, brother and uncle were inside, I've often been celebrated for breaking the cycle. A few weeks ago, there was a British-Jamaican man in my class whose dad and brother had also been inside. I looked at him and imagined what it would be like if I had told people that my family had been in jail and I was black. I expect people would think they needed to keep an eye on me.

Stepping into prison reminds me of my own background, but it also reminds me that I escaped my background, and that I would have had fewer escape routes available to me had I not been white.

*

Eighteen months ago, only two students showed up to my class. Rocky was mixed-race and had 'HMP Soldier' tattooed on his neck. Emmanuel was white and had long hair and a braided goatee. He wore a set of purple rosary beads around his wrist.

I looked in the corridor to see if anyone else was coming. A young black man was arguing with a black officer who had put him on basic.

'Sell-out,' the young man said and walked away.

I waited another ten minutes to see if anyone else arrived, but I heard there had been a fight on one of the wings and men were being kept in their cells. I closed the door to get on with the lesson.

I wrote at the top of the whiteboard, 'The different kinds of animals'.

Below I wrote a taxonomy of animals from Jorge Luis Borges's fictitious, ancient Chinese encyclopaedia called 'Celestial Emporium of Benevolent Knowledge'. 'Those that belong to the emperor. Embalmed ones. Those that are trained. Suckling pigs. Mermaids. Stray dogs. Those that are included in this classification. Those that tremble as if they were mad.'

'What's your star sign?' Emmanuel asked me.

'I don't have one,' I said.

'You're so sarcastic. You might be a Capricorn.'

I continued writing the list: 'Innumerable ones. Those drawn with a very fine camel-hair brush.'

'Where are you from, Andy?' Rocky asked.

'I was born in England,' I said.

'But you're not completely English,' he said.

'Both my parents were born in England. So were their parents.'

Outside, I hardly ever get asked where I am from. In prison, I'm asked a few times a week. It's sometimes because my students of colour would like to hear that I'm not completely white. Also, because everyone here keeps themselves to themselves, nobody ever finds out who anybody else really is. What you are becomes the substitute for who you are.

I turned back to the board and kept writing: 'Those that have just broken the flower vase. Those that, at a distance, resemble flies.'

'Do you just love the sunbed then?' Rocky said. He winked at me.

'My great-great-grandparents were Romany travellers. But they settled in the East End,' I said.

'I saw a documentary about Romanies last week.'

'Then you know more about them than I do,' I said.

'I knew you was a little bit something else.' He looked pleased.

I point to the list on the board. 'What do you th—'

'When were you born, Andy?' Emmanuel asked.

'In the morning,' I said.

Emmanuel scowled at me.

The door banged open. A man charged in and ran to the corner of the room. His cheeks, forehead and hairline were marked with scars. His face looked like a page of writing.

'Hello,' I said.

He ignored me and watched the door.

'This is philosophy,' I said.

He looked me up and down and then looked back at the door.

'Do you want to have a seat?' I said.

'A screw is after me.'

'Look, we're just starting the lesson. Take a seat. If the officer comes, I'll ask them if I can keep you in my class,' I said.

He laughed at me.

'How many times you been stopped and searched?' he asked.

Emmanuel watched me. He twiddled the ends of his hair.

'You've never been stopped and searched, have you?' the man said.

'I have.'

'Did they write you up? I bet they did. I bet they called you sir, too. "Oh, sorry for bothering you, sir."'

'I can't remember. It was a long time ago,' I said.

'Of course it was.'

He ran across the room and out of the door. I went to the doorway and watched him sprint down the corridor and duck into another classroom. I closed the door halfway, but I felt strange and I opened it again.

'He might come back,' I said.

'That is such a Capricorn thing to say,' Emmanuel said.

When I was eighteen, I was walking along an empty A-road at 2 a.m. by myself, coming back from a friend's house. I was wearing a dark grey hoodie and a black scarf that covered my nose. A police car pulled over in front of me. The officers got out and asked me questions about where I had been and where I was going. They told me they were going to conduct a stop and search.

'I haven't done anything,' I said.

The officers told me to turn out my pockets and hold my arms out.

I did as they said. They went through my pockets. I turned my head away and acted aloof, but one of my knees kept trembling.

They found nothing on me, but I felt no vindication.

'I haven't done anything. Breathalyse me if you want. It will come up zero,' I said.

The officers got back in their car and drove off.

I walked home, feeling guilty. The executioner in my head told me that the police wouldn't have stopped me unless I'd done something wrong. The police know something about me that I don't. Next time they'll take me to the station.

I got home, took off my hoodie and chucked it in the bottom of my wardrobe.

A couple of days after, I was in a charity shop and bought a navy-blue linen jacket. It was still winter, so I could only wear it when I wore my thick red woolly jumper underneath. I had to pull the jacket on tightly over the jumper. It pinched at the armpits.

Two weeks later, I was walking home in the early hours of the morning, wearing my red woolly jumper and blue linen jacket. A police car pulled up alongside me. I felt dread. I tried to resign myself to whatever they were going to do with me.

They wound down their window. I crouched down to look inside and saw a male and a female officer. They looked at me and then glanced at each other.

'Aww,' the female officer said.

The police car pulled away and drove off.

*

If I had been black, I think it's less likely the officer would have said 'Aww.' I doubt that changing my clothes would have been enough to change the way I was seen.

In *The Wretched of the Earth*, the philosopher Frantz Fanon wrote, 'Confronted with a world configured by the coloniser, the colonised subject is always presumed guilty. The colonised subject does not accept his guilt, but rather considers it a kind of curse, a sword of Damocles.' In the ancient Greek myth, Damocles lived every day with a sword hanging by a thread above his head, knowing it could drop on him at any time. Fanon was describing what it's like to live with an executioner.

Every day at 5 p.m. I walk through the landing on my way out of the prison. I see the number of black and brown people being locked up for the night and I'm reminded that there are executioners that aren't only a voice in the head.

Today, I run another session on Malcolm X and we touch on how X's preoccupation with being emasculated would have had something to do with the fact that he was living in a time where white Americans would have called him 'Boy'. At the end of the class, a couple of the black students ask me if we can talk about philosophy and race in the next session. There is enough trust and openness in the group for that to sound like a good idea.

I'm interested to talk about race too. When I was younger, I didn't fully appreciate how my race had shaped my life the way it had. I didn't see a huge amount of difference between the oppression people of colour suffered from the criminal justice system, and the police trying to arrest my brother two hours after he'd been released from prison. But as I've got older and my experience has become broader, I see how if

Jason had been black or brown the odds are that he would have been arrested even more and received tougher sentences. I'm curious to understand these realities of race more. At the same time, I remember Paul gazing at me from across the table at Chloe's dinner party and what it felt like to be looked at with curiosity. I hope to be interested in the men's ideas without looking at them as Paul looked at me.

On Saturday, I sit at my desk trying to prepare something, looking for ideas in the pages of books by Toni Morrison, George Schuyler and Kwame Anthony Appiah. I feel lost. I left university in 2009 having not discussed race at all. We didn't study a single person of colour, but we did look at plenty of thinkers from the western canon who said that non-Europeans were incapable of reason and innately inferior. I think about my nan's house. She leaves her front door open in the afternoon so that her British-Pakistani neighbour Hana can let herself in. They sit in the living room, drink sugary tea and complain about the housing officer who never picks up the phone, social services meddling in everyone's business, the Percy Ingle bakery that has closed because of gentrification and how the police nick people when it's not necessary and fail to nick them when it is. They talk almost exclusively in stories, taking it in turns to be each other's audience, as the other tells about what happened on the street last week or forty years ago. When Hana talks, Nan often nods along, but at certain points she can only listen. I don't mean to sound romantic; I know there's plenty of racism in working-class communities, but as I try to plan my lesson it strikes me how I find it easier to talk about race on an East London council estate than I did in my university seminars.

I manage to put together something on Audre Lorde's

essay 'The Uses of Anger'. On Monday morning, I'm in my classroom looking over my lesson plan. The students arrive, but the two men who wanted me to run the class are not here. They have been transferred. I have two new students. The first is a middle-aged white man called Seb. His file says he's in for crimes to do with right-wing extremism. The second is an Eritrean man called Nebay. He only knows a handful of English phrases, most of which are about life on the landing, like 'bang up', 'canteen' and 'phone call.' He was supposed to be in the English class but it's full, so he's been put in here instead.

Suddenly I'm standing before a very different group to the one that wanted me to run a session on the philosophy of race. Seb often complains to my colleague that he's a victim of racism, claiming that he's an ethnic minority on his landing and that the black officers treat him unfairly compared to how they treat black prisoners. Beginning a discussion on 'The Uses of Anger' could either be the best or worst thing to do right now, but I decide to put my lesson plan away. I hope to get it out again soon.

I look through an old file in the corner of the room, find some English worksheets and give one to Nebay.

It's now the middle of the Covid pandemic. Six months after I put my 'The Uses of Anger' lesson plan away, prisons went into lockdown and I haven't been able to run that class. It could be a year before I'll be able to go back and teach inside. I'm disappointed that I didn't get to have that discussion.

I email three people who were once held inside, but now work in prisons – Mandy Ogunmokun, Jamal Khan and Brenda Birungi. I tell them I'm writing a memoir about prison and that I want it to include a philosophical discussion about race where readers can see the different opinions of people who've been inside. They agree and we arrange to meet together online.

Mandy used to struggle with addiction and was in and out of prison every year for twenty years. She says that going to jail was a relief. She often felt more safe and free inside than she did outside. Prison was like her home. After her recovery, she became a drug worker in jails and set up a charity called Treasures Foundation to provide housing to women who have been released from prison. Mandy lived with the women, teaching them how to cook, clean and look after the plants. After several years, she moved out and some of the people she'd nurtured took her role, helping new women who had come out of prison to make a home.

Jamal grew up in poverty and was taken into care when he was a child. He witnessed a lot of violence in his community, including seeing his childhood friend shot dead in front of him. Jamal was excluded from school and when he was fifteen he was given a five-year prison sentence. He felt like his life was over. In his cell, he began journaling, writing poems and short stories. It became a form of therapy to make sense of everything he'd been through. After being released he won the Waterstones Emerging Young Writers Award. He currently works with a charity called No More Exclusions and runs writing workshops with young people in his community who are going through the same kinds of experiences he went through when he was a teenager.

Brenda was born in Uganda and came to the UK as a baby. When she was convicted at twenty-one, the authorities told her that she was going to be deported to Africa. She told them that she had a British passport. They put her in a van and sent her to a detention centre for foreign nationals. A black officer opened the gate to let her in. After that she saw no more black officers in the jail. She wrote a letter to the governors to explain that there had been some sort of mistake, but a few days later she was given her deportation date. She wondered if she had spelt some words wrong in her letter and that had made the people in the office think she wasn't really British. In her cell she went through the dictionary, checking the spelling in her letter.

Brenda remembered an old photo that she had lost a few years before. It was taken when she was five and all the children in her south London primary school were dressed up in costume for Victorians Day. It shows Brenda standing alongside the other children, wearing a white pinny and frilly bonnet. She wished she knew where that photo was now. Her mother offered to send her in some things from home, including some CDs. 'Don't send any Ugandan music,' Brenda said. 'I don't want to give them any reason to think they can put me on that plane.'

The prison was in the countryside. In the exercise yard, the air smelt of manure. When Brenda covered her nose, some of the officers laughed at her and said, 'What's wrong?'

'What do you mean what's wrong? Can't you smell that smell?' she said.

'It doesn't smell. You don't know what fresh air smells like where you're from.'

She looked at the guards who were unaffected by the stench and wondered if they were right, that this is what fresh air smells like.

Brenda complained about how small the portions of food were. One officer said to her, 'Are you saying that you get three meals a day where you come from?' Unlike in regular jails, people in the foreign national prison were allowed keys to their own cell. When the officers handed Brenda her key, she felt like she was being mocked – being given a symbol of freedom whilst having her actual freedom taken from her.

Eventually, she was able to convince the authorities she was British, and it was arranged for her to serve the rest of her sentence in a regular prison. When a female officer from London escorted Brenda out of the gates of the foreign national prison, the officer smelt the manure, covered her nose and said 'Urgh.'

'You can smell that too, right?' Brenda said.

'Smell it? It stinks,' the officer said.

'Thank you!' Brenda said.

Brenda was driven to the regular prison. Free from the fear of being deported, she focused on writing. Since her release she has been working as Lady Unchained – a spoken-word artist, poetry teacher and radio broadcaster. Recently, she visited some prisons in Uganda, taking food and clothes for the people inside. They looked at her and muttered to each other, 'What's this British woman doing here?'

We all log on and say hello. 'I'm writing about prison through the lens of having had a dad, brother and uncle who were inside,' I say. 'But my family's story is a white working-class one. I know there are lots of other stories in prison too.'

'When your brother was in jail, when you was a kid, did you talk about it with anyone?' Brenda asks me.

'Not really.'

'That was the same with my nephew. He'd visit me, but when he went back home he wouldn't talk about it.'

'That's common, huh?'

Brenda nods.

Mandy says, 'Shame gets passed down. Families pass it down to their children. The children feel ashamed but they can't even tell what they've done wrong.'

I blink.

'I still have to work with that,' she says. 'I still have a punisher in my head.'

A few minutes later, the discussion is underway. 'The philosopher Audre Lorde thought that anger could have revolutionary potential,' I say. 'In "The Uses of Anger", she said that every day black women in America have reason to feel rage, but fear that expressing it will see them condemned as the angry black woman. Instead, many black women become apologetic and guilty about who they are, but Lorde said that guilt was corrosive. "I have no creative use for guilt, yours or my own. Guilt is only another way of avoiding informed action, of buying time out of the pressing need to make clear choices, out of the approaching storm that can feed the earth as well as bend the trees."'

'I'm mixed race and I was born in the sixties,' Mandy says. 'My mum was a prostitute. My dad was a punter. My grandmother was my mum's pimp. And that's how I came about. Growing up, I saw people staring at me and just thought there was something wrong with me. I hated my black side, only I didn't know it. I didn't know I was brainwashed to think there was something wrong with my colour. Even my grandmother used to call me and my sister n****rs, and she was one of the ones who actually loved us.'

As I listen to Mandy's story, I see the differences between the punisher in her head and the one in mine. The executioner in my head has never told me I should hate myself because of my race. My shame plays out privately rather than through people staring at me on the street.

Mandy continues, 'I became a prostitute, thief and a drug addict. I slept with a heroin syringe under my pillow. I was in and out of Holloway prison for twenty years. After I went through recovery, I went back to Holloway to give a talk for Black History Month. I was reading something from Martin Luther King and I broke down crying. It was the speech where he says that one day he dreams of black and white living together in harmony. All my life, one part of me had been hating the other. I wasn't living in harmony with myself. That's what had kept me imprisoned. I just cried and cried.'

I say, 'Lorde said it is better to embrace anger than to feel guilty, but also said there is a difference between living in a cacophony and symphony of anger. Black women, she said, "have had to learn to orchestrate those furies so that they do not tear us apart. We have had to learn to move through them and use them for strength and force and insight in our daily lives."'

Mandy says, 'Before my recovery, my head was always full of the noise of trauma. It was that harsh, discordant life that Audre talks about. Nobody would ever listen to me because whenever I tried to get my point across, I was just rage.'

'But today,' she says, 'everything that's happened to me in my past, every single drop has been turned into something

I'm using in the present. I'm working with women who've been through the same trauma and been in and out of prison like me. I battle with them side by side, not in a controlling way, but letting them know that I'm here and that change is possible. Sometimes they think there's no hope, and I tell them to hang on, just hang on a little bit longer. Nothing I've been through has been wasted. All that noise has come together into something positive. The cacophony has become a symphony – it's like Audre says, I can move. I can move.'

I say, 'Lorde believed in the transformative power of anger. She wrote, "I have suckled the wolf's lip of anger and I have used it for illumination, laughter, protection, fire in places where there was no light, no food, no sisters, no quarter."'

'Anger can illuminate,' Jamal says. 'In court, none of what I'd been through in my childhood was taken into account. I sat there and didn't say much. When they sentenced me, I was so angry how my personal situation had been overlooked. But that anger was useful, because it showed me that the system wasn't gonna help me turn my life around. I was going to have to do that myself. In jail I started writing my story, telling it how it should be told rather than how it was told in court. Articulating myself illuminated things for me. And ultimately it led to a brighter future.'

'Do you think Lorde is right that anger can bring protection?' I ask.

Brenda says, 'When I was in prison, what I most needed protection from was my anger at myself.'

Jamal and Mandy nod.

'There's anger that gives you the energy to create change and there's anger that makes you feel powerless and trapped,'

Jamal says. 'When I came out of prison, I was doing a lot of spoken-word events, speaking about my experience. Everything I was writing was about injustice. My whole identity was based around being someone who was impacted by the criminal justice system. That's who I was.

'The poet Ebonee Davis wrote, "So many people are actually afraid to heal because their entire identity is centred around the trauma they've experienced. They have no idea who they are outside of that trauma. And this unknown can be terrifying." That was me. I was so caught up in my past. I had to question if it was giving me any joy. I decided to move forward from that. Rather than talk about the system which we know is wrong, I wanted to build towards a better system. I came off stage and started supporting young people who've been through what I've been through and need help.

'That's not easy, specifically for people who have been released from prison and make a living out of their experience of being inside. That's what they depend on. But I had to if I was going to move beyond my anger and do something that truly gives me joy.'

I say, 'Another philosopher, Minna Salami, reflects on the difference between joy and anger as a means of resistance. She says that people from marginalized groups are burdened by always having to explain themselves, unlike most middle-class white men. If you're black or brown, it's as if your identity is some kind of "crime scene". Salami says that in response, marginalized groups use things like Black Power to "take up arms", and use their identity as a "weapon" for empowerment. Whilst she thinks that this has been successful in many ways, it also keeps the oppressor at the centre of the story. The weapon is always pointed at him.'

Jamal nods.

I say, 'Salami focuses less on black power and more on black joy. Joy gives no status to the oppressor.'

Brenda says, 'Before I went to prison, whenever I used to talk about racism or slavery, I always used to apologize beforehand, like how white people sometimes apologize just before they're about to say something racist. I never wanted to speak Luganda in public. I'd let people assume I was Jamaican. Whenever the fact I'm African came up, I would be like, "Let's move on, we don't need to talk about it." I saw my own heritage as white people saw it. As a kid, Africa to me was Comic Relief; starving children with flies on them. I thought you only went there if you'd committed a crime.

'But in a strange way, going to prison gave me a new-found confidence in my heritage. I feel a joy about being African I never had before. Now when I perform poems about slavery and racism I don't apologize for doing that. Now, I do talk Luganda in public. When people say I'm Jamaican I tell them that actually I'm African. I'm flying to Uganda again in three weeks and I can't wait.'

'That sounds like it could so easily have gone the other way,' I say. 'For many people, going to prison reaffirms their shame.'

'It was through embracing my anger that I embraced who I really am.'

We discuss whether anger or joy is the better means of resistance and Mandy shares another story.

'When I started going into Holloway as a worker, I'd see

this officer and say, "Hello. Good Morning." She would just completely blank me. Every day, I went in. She'd blank me. I'd say "Hello." "Good Morning." "Isn't it a beautiful morning."'

'That's so defiant,' Jamal says.

Mandy says, 'Then one day, she said hello back. She started trying to have a conversation with me. But inside I'm thinking, I don't wanna talk to you. I only want to say good morning.'

We all laugh.

'I had to work at talking with her,' Mandy says. 'After a few weeks, I realized she was human and she had problems too.'

One reason I didn't tell anyone Jason was in prison when I was a kid was because I feared I'd somehow be in trouble. People would assume my brother was bad and therefore that I was bad too. I kept my mouth shut and tried not to look conspicuous. I think of how Brenda's nephew didn't talk about it either. I wonder if his sense of punishment by association might have been even more intense than mine. If it had been the case that my brother faced deportation because of the colour of his skin or the sound of his surname, I might have feared that the basic fact of my skin or my surname could mean trouble for me too.

'I used to be an inmate in Downview prison,' Brenda says, 'and then ten years later I went in as a facilitator to run a class on poetry. They asked me if once I finished my workshop did I want to be taken on a tour and see my old cell. I was so excited. I couldn't wait to see the cell where I started writing and where things started to come together that led me to coming back here, not as an inmate but as a teacher.

'So after my class, I was walking through the prison yard with two white ladies either side of me – my producer and the woman who had booked us to come in – and a big, massive white officer stops me and says, "Why aren't you back on the landing? You should be in your cell."

'"Pardon," I said.

'"You should be back in your cell," he said.

'The two white women with me explained to him that I'm not a prisoner I'm a visiting poet. The officer went red. He didn't apologize, he just went bright red. I just said, "Oh, you think I'm an inmate. No, no. I'm just here to facilitate."

'After we left the prison, my producer was so angry and she wished I could get angry too, but she also knew that it's more complicated for me as a black woman. It made her sad, but I felt so much power saying, "Oh no, I'm here to facilitate." If I'd have got angry I would have had to carry that anger all the way home into the next day, thinking why did that officer speak like that to me, I thought I was doing so well. How dare he. But instead, I went home with the joy that once upon a time, the system took power away from me, but look at me now.'

Inside

> There is no point in staying stuck . . . But there is even less point in pretending to be free. I feel on the verge of a great transformation which may be as simple as becoming interested in other things.
>
> EDWARD ST AUBYN

A week after Nebay was put in my class, he's still coming. I've given him almost all the worksheets from the file at the back of the room. Today I give him one called, 'We're going on holiday'. The rest of the class discuss Epictetus's definition of freedom.

Twenty minutes before the end of the session, the English teacher comes in and tells Nebay that he will be joining her class now. Nebay packs up his things. We say goodbye and he leaves.

The following morning, I take a photo of the oven and leave home. Ten minutes later, I cross the road and I fear I've left the gas on. I look at the photo I took, but it doesn't put me at ease. I think, 'What if I took the photo and then switched the stove back on by accident,' as if I can't be sure that I don't have an evil hand that does things while I'm not watching. I turn around, cross the road again and run back home to check and see that I have not left the gas on.

An hour later, I walk into the reception of a high-security prison and the sensor picks up my body passing through the door, triggering an automated announcement: 'Stop! It is illegal to bring mobile phones into the establishment. If you are found to be in possession of a mobile phone inside the establishment, you will be prosecuted.'

I reach into my rucksack and take out my passport, chewing gum and other contraband items and put them in a locker. Somebody else walks into reception and the announcement sounds again. 'Stop! It is illegal to bring mobile phones into the establishment. If you are found to be in possession of a mobile phone inside the establishment, you will be prosecuted.'

I take my phone out of my pocket, send my mother a message and sign off with two kisses and wait for the second tick to say that the message has been delivered. I put my phone in the locker, turn the key and put it in my pocket.

Another person walks through the door and triggers the sensor. The announcement sounds. I pat down all the pockets of my trousers and coat to check I really have put my phone inside the locker. I can't feel my phone, but I think, what if it has fallen into the lining of my coat, somewhere I wouldn't be able to easily find it?

I open the locker. My phone is there. I pick it up and check social media to see if the woman I have a crush on has liked something I posted an hour ago. She hasn't.

'. . . you will be prosecuted,' the voice above says.

I put my phone in my locker. I touch it with my hand to confirm that it is in my locker. I look in my bag, somehow needing to check that my phone is not in two places at once. I shut the locker and go into the security room.

The door behind me shuts and I join the queue to be searched. On the wall, there is a mugshot of a former security officer. She bought second-hand smartphones off the internet for £250 and sold them to men inside for around £1,500. She got arrested and sentenced to several years of prison time. I must have my phone on me somewhere, I think. It's somewhere I can't find, but it's definitely on me. I want to turn back, but it's too late. The officer calls me towards him.

I step forward. The officer searches me. He doesn't find a phone.

This prison has a Body Orifice Security Scanner, also known as a BOSS chair. When you sit in it, it can detect metal inside the vagina or rectum. I'm disappointed that the officer doesn't ask me to sit in it today, since the BOSS chair is the one part of prison security that doesn't make me anxious. Even in my most intense panics, I'm confident I haven't unknowingly put my iPhone inside my anus.

Despite such intimate levels of security, illegal smartphones are still common in prison. The LONG-CZ phone has become a popular choice on the landing. It's small enough to store inside your ass, and it is made of plastic. The BOSS chair can't detect it.

A minute later, I walk down the landing. I automatically put my hand in my pocket to check my messages, but it is empty. I feel bereft that I cannot scroll through social media or check to see if my icons have little red notification dots next to them. But by 10 a.m. it feels nice not to have a phone. My mind feels clearer now that it's not being pillaged by pings and alerts. But being disconnected is an uneasy pleasure whilst I'm in here. As I cross men on the stairway, I enjoy the absence of weight in my pocket, but some of them will have a phone in their rectum.

Half an hour later, I'm teaching in a room usually used

for workshops, where men would ordinarily pack teabags, UHT milk and sugar into small plastic bags that will go to youth jails. Unlike my classroom, there's a phone in here, mounted on the wall in the corner of the room. During the class, the men sit in a circle and discuss questions of free will, responsibility and fate. One man goes into the corner to make a ninety-second call to his daughter. Another man phones his solicitor.

At 1 p.m. I go through security and unlock my locker. I step out of reception, look at my phone and a list of notifications glows on the screen. The voice saying 'You will be prosecuted' fades away behind me.

When I was eighteen, I read Franz Kafka's fiction for the first time. It was a story called *In the Penal Colony*, about a man who was accused of a crime, though he didn't know what he had done wrong. In that world the accused were assumed to be guilty and never allowed to defend themselves. He had been placed in an apparatus where a device would carve his crime on his back, inscribing the words into his skin over and over again until he bled to death. I finished reading the story but kept the book in my hand, absorbing the dark resonance of it. Kafka had managed to communicate a mood that until that point I had felt alone with: that it's too late. The condemned man is already in the apparatus before the story even starts; by the time he makes his first appearance, all of his chances have already expired. I turned to the back cover and looked at the photo of Kafka. He had the same sticky-out ears and adolescent frame as me. I wondered who this man was.

As I read more over the next few weeks, I found out that

when Kafka was a child, he was physically and emotionally abused by his father. It left the young Kafka terrified and ashamed. He went on to write numerous stories about the nightmare of arbitrary condemnation, where a man is helpless before a malevolent authority. He'd become a specialist in the executioner. When he was thirty-five, he wrote a letter to his father telling him, 'My writing was all about you; all I did there, after all, was to bemoan what I could not bemoan upon your breast.' Perhaps he was referring to his story *The Judgement*, where a father orders his adult son to go and drown himself and the son complies.

For that summer, I was obsessed with Kafka. On the hottest day of the year, I sat reading him on a bench in the park, laughing out loud at his deadpan absurdity. My then-girlfriend Jess and I went to an expensive hotel for the weekend, one with sex toys on the menu. In the morning, I sat up in bed underlining Kafka's sentences in green pen. I believed that Kafka would make me feel less alone with the executioner. When Jessica and I got back from our weekend, she broke up with me.

For the last fifteen years, my affinity to Kafka has been as troubling as it has been reassuring. The more I've got to know his work, the more I think he seemed to write as a kind of anti-therapy, sitting at his desk at 2 a.m., always returning to the same type of story about men who never escape the father, the law, the executioner. It was as though he had given up on escape and settled for the illusion of control his pen could give him instead, the omnipotent author writing the same fatalistic story over and over. Reading him, I'm no longer alone with the executioner, but instead I'm in the company of a strange man who knows his torture so intimately because he is the one inflicting much of it on himself. I worry that the years I've spent reading Kafka have made the executioner in my head more powerful by endowing him with literary apparatus. Am I using Kafka's masochism to enact my own?

I also try to control the executioner. I check my locker several times to see if my phone is in there, return home to make sure I haven't burnt the house down and go back through my every move to make sure the executioner doesn't have anything on me. I also reread Kafka's stories to see a controlled performance of my own nightmare. The book I return to the most is *The Trial*. It's about a man called Joseph K., who wakes up on the morning of his thirtieth birthday to find two officials in his room. They tell him he is under arrest. He asks them what he is being arrested for. The two men tell him that he is requested to go to his trial on Sunday. K. asks them again what he has done. The officials repeat that he must go to his trial and they leave.

Later that day, K.'s friends invite him to a party on a boat happening on Sunday, but when Sunday comes, he decides to go to his hearing instead. Since the officials didn't give him a time, he decides he should get to the courthouse for 9 a.m., as soon as it opens. K. leaves his house and runs to make sure he doesn't arrive late.

He comes to a suburban street and through a window in one of the houses, he sees a man holding a small baby.

K. pauses and looks around.

Through the window of another house, he sees a man savouring a cigarette. On the street, a fruitmonger works behind their stall. Two friends are having a conversation across the road from one another and laughing.

K. turns and goes to his trial.

He returns to his hearing each Sunday until eventually he is executed. He never finds out what he was guilty of.

I return home from the high-security prison. At 3 p.m. I'm sitting on a bench in my garden. Small white jasmine flowers creep up the wall. I close my eyes to better enjoy the feeling of the sun on my arms. A subtle feeling of doom intrudes. I think how awful it would be if when I went into prison this morning I accidentally took my phone in and accidentally left it there. I know this is an absurd thought since I used my phone only an hour ago and it is now charging in my bedroom. But I think, what if an officer finds my phone inside. I'd be arrested the next time I went into work.

I take a deep breath, inhaling the scent of jasmine, and I try to dismiss my thoughts. But the feeling that I must have done something wrong won't leave me.

I stand up, walk into the house and go up the stairs. I open my bedroom door and see my phone on my desk. I pick it up and squeeze it until my fingertips turn white.

'Fuck,' I say.

I left the garden just as Joseph K. turned away from the street. I've just run to the executioner.

A few days later, I step into the reception of another prison. It's not a high-security institution, so instead of the overhead announcements and body scanners, there's just a large sign that says, 'If you're found with a mobile phone inside the establishment, WE WILL CALL THE POLICE.' I don't know when this started, but I've come to find this sign reassuring. The executioner so often makes me distrust my senses; the sight of an authoritarian message threatening legal action against me makes it seem like my setting is almost harmonious with my mind.

I put my phone, chewing gum and passport inside a locker. I turn and step towards the security door. I think, 'What if my phone is in my bag.' I check my bag, and my phone is not there. I think, 'What if it's in my bag but I can't see it.'

'For fuck's sake,' I say.

The officer behind the desk looks at me.

I turn around and walk back to my locker and open it. I see my phone inside. I'm angry that I have just run to the executioner's call again. Yet I can't shake the fear. I search my bag for my phone, whilst I'm able to see my phone in my locker.

The officer watches me.

I lock my phone away, take a deep breath and go into the prison. On the landing, I see a man wearing a yellow and green jumpsuit, or an 'escape suit' as it is known here. Men have to wear them if they are deemed an escape risk. If they did get away, then they would be easy to spot in a crowd. In one cell, a man is staging a dirty protest. His door is half open. A smell like sewage hits me and I quicken my walk. The man locked in the cell next to his is banging on his door and shouting at his neighbour to pack it in.

I set up my classroom. Andros is the first to arrive, a short, wiry man who always wears the sleeves of his tracksuit top pushed up to his elbows. His accent switches between cockney and the multicultural London English that young working-class people in the city speak today. When he says 'thing' he sometimes goes 'fing' and other times goes 'ting'. He talks with the old blokes on the wing as easily as he talks to the teenagers. He recently put in for a transfer to a lower-security prison where there are showers and phones in the cells, but his request got refused because Andros's younger brother is in that prison. It's not against the rules for siblings to jail together; some share cells. But Andros's brother works in that prison, as part of a rehabilitation project. If he and Andros were in the same prison it would be classed as a conflict of interest.

Andros walks over to my whiteboard and tuts at how dirty it is. He picks up a cloth and spray – and wipes the board down.

This is the second year Andros is doing my course. After he finished his first course with me, he asked if he could do it again. I told him that the lessons would all be the same, but he said he wanted to do it anyway. 'They'll put me in the maths class otherwise. I've passed that course four times already.'

He wipes the board until it looks as good as new. He puts the spray and cloth down. He holds his lower back and groans. 'The mattresses in this place. I'm getting too old for prison,' he says.

Andros is nearly forty. Last week he told me he'd heard people on the radio saying that prisons aren't necessary and we should abolish them. 'Where would they put all of us? Have they thought about that?' he told me. 'So they think they can just show up and click their fingers and say, OK, no more prison? They don't have a clue.' It reminded me of my brother. Jason has a similar almost-offended response to abolitionism. I think he sees it as a denial of the kind of life he's had; I see it as a way in which he and I could have spent more of our lives together.

The rest of the men arrive and I get the class underway.

'Imagine a prisoner who is happy in his cell. He has no desire to leave,' I say.

'Because he's playing on his smartphone?' Andros says.

'Is that man free?' I ask.

Andros says, 'No. Man is in a cell.' A few minutes later he says, 'Or maybe, yeah, man is as free as he wants to be.' A moment later he asks, 'I don't get this guy. If man doesn't want to be free then is he free?'

'What do you think?' I ask.

Andros opens his mouth but hesitates.

'Bastard,' he says.

The men laugh.

I tell the class about aporia – an ancient Greek word meaning 'without a path'. Aporia is a state of mind you arrive at in a philosophical dialogue where you realize your basic beliefs and assumptions might not be true. The path you were walking along has come to a stop and you're unsure what to think next. All of a sudden you are stranded. But from that state of confusion you have the chance to truly think for yourself and carve out your path moving forward.

'That's it,' Andros says. 'You're always aporiaing me. Why you gotta be like that, Andy.'

The men laugh again.

I feel awkward talking to them about the value of uncertainty when I remember how I squeezed my phone until my fingertips went white. I'm asking them to allow themselves to become stranded, whilst I keep taking the same path to the executioner.

An hour later, an officer shouts, 'Free flow!' Three or four men gather round Taff to shake his hand and wish him luck.

Taff is in his early thirties and has a cosmopolitan-sounding accent from where he went to various international schools around the world as a kid. This is his first time inside. He was jailed a few weeks after his wife gave birth to their first child, but tomorrow he'll be released to do the last few months of his sentence wearing an electronic tag.

'Eat a McDonald's for me,' Andros says.

Andros often says this to me as well. Sometimes, at 5 p.m., when he sees me walking down the landing with my coat on, about to leave the prison, he fist bumps me and says, 'Eat a McDonald's for me,' or 'Eat a delicious meal for me tonight, OK?' I always laugh awkwardly. I don't know what to say back.

'I've been dreaming about food for months,' Taff says. 'When I first got here, I thought the first thing I'm going to do when I get home is sleep. But now I'm not sure how I'm gonna be able to get to sleep unless I can hear a fight going on in the next room. I'm going to ask my wife to kick the living room wall until she hears me start snoring.'

Andros says, 'I just cried the last time I got out. The whole two and a half years I was in jail, I never cried once. But on the first night in my hostel, I sat on the end of the bed and cried.'

After the class, I'm on my way out of the prison and an officer tells me to join a line. They are conducting a spontaneous search of everyone. I get to the front of the queue. An officer searches me. I know my phone is in my locker but it's still a relief when he doesn't find it in my pockets.

The following afternoon, I'm in Jason's living room. My brother is in Scott's room trying to get him off his Xbox so we can go out. I wait next to a standing lamp that's plugged into the wall. The switch on the wall socket is not turned off. Neither are the switches connecting the TV socket.

Fifteen years ago, Jason would have to turn off every switch in the house or else he couldn't sleep. When he adjusted the TV volume by two units, he'd do it by going up by four markers then down by two. He had to open and shut a door three times every time he walked through one. It could take him forty minutes to iron a pair of shorts before he was satisfied that both legs were equally smooth. Sometimes he still needs things to be a certain way in order to relax, but he's nowhere near as bad as he used to be.

During his worst period of anxiety, Jason and a friend were burgling a college in the middle of the night. They gathered up as many DVD players as they could carry from the top-floor classrooms and carried them downstairs to the foyer, where they saw four police officers waiting for them. My brother dropped the DVD players, ran down the foyer and towards a corridor that would lead him out of the building. The police chased him. Jason sprinted down the corridor, pushed open the door to the exit and continued running.

He shouted, 'Fuck sake!' He turned around, ran back to open and shut the door three times.

He opened the door. Two police officers pushed him to the ground, put his hands behind his back and handcuffed him.

I go into Jason's kitchen and pour myself a cup of water. I feel the breeze on my arms from the ajar window. I bring the cup to my lips.

An alert pings on my phone. I look at it and see a notification reporting a breaking story about how several men have been caught attempting to escape HMP Winchester.

Jason comes in the kitchen wearing a new T-shirt with a tag still attached to the neckline. He opens a drawer and rummages for some scissors.

'Apparently some people tried to escape from Winchester prison last night,' I say.

Jason closes one drawer and opens another.

'They didn't succeed,' I say.

He grabs some scissors out of the drawer, hands them to me and turns around. I cut the tag from the neckline of his shirt.

'Let's go,' he says.

We set off to the park with Scott and Dean. Scott is now ten and Dean is five. Jason stops to catch up with an old mate of his who is sat begging outside Tesco. Bored of the grown-ups talking, Scott and Dean play rock-paper-scissors with each other. A few minutes later, we get to the park. Tall stone sculptures of various dinosaurs are positioned throughout the field. It's almost thirty degrees. Jason puts his hand inside the sleeve of his T-shirt and scratches his shoulder, revealing a scar on his bicep. It's blobby-looking, like it was made by something blunt and forceful, like a screwdriver rather than a knife.

'Where did you get that scar?' I ask.

'Oh,' he says. 'It was—'

Scott and Dean race up to him screaming and throw their arms around his torso.

'I won,' Dean says.

'No, I won,' Scott says.

They laugh hard and try to catch their breath. Jason strokes their heads.

'It was years ago, Bruv,' Jason says to me.

I give him a sheepish smile.

The two boys run off towards a stone dinosaur. Jason and I walk in their trail. Jason smokes a roll-up. He keeps turning his face away from me to blow out his smoke.

'How are you, Bruv? You look tired,' Jason says.

'I've been working a lot,' I say.

'I worry about you going into prison.'

'I'm fine.'

'Does it ever affect your mental health?' he asks.

I shrug. 'It's not like how it was for you.'

He screws his face up and looks away. I know he finds my guilt intense and patronizing. I wish I knew how to stop it.

We walk past a rose bush and I catch the scent of one of the flowers. I feel melancholy that this day is passing me by.

Jason looks back at me.

'You could do so many things with your life,' he says. 'Why prison? Is it cos of me? It affected you when I went away, didn't it?'

'It's what I want to do,' I say.

He gives me a sad smile.

'Are you happy doing it?' he asks.

'I don't really think about it that way,' I say.

'I want you to be happy, Andy.'

I look down at my feet.

Scott points at a stone diplodocus with a long grey neck and runs up to it. Dean follows him. Jason asks me to take a photo, and he goes and stands in front of the diplodocus with his arm around his two sons. I step back and point my phone at them.

Jason nudges Scott and tells him to smile.

A notification appears at the top of my screen. It's about HMP Winchester.

'Cheese!' the boys say.

I open the notification. The article says that men used plastic knives and forks to dig tunnels through the prison's crumbling walls.

'Hurry up, Bruv,' Jason says. 'My face is hurting.'

The next day, I head back to the prison where we said goodbye to Taff. I enter reception and see the sign that says, 'If you're found with a mobile phone inside the establishment, WE WILL CALL THE POLICE.' I put my prohibited items in a locker and go into the prison.

Thirty minutes later, I'm setting the chairs up around the large table in the middle of my classroom. I put one less seat out now that Taff is not here. An officer in the corridor hollers, 'Free flow.'

I'm at my desk making notes when Andros comes in. I glance up but keep on writing. Andros picks up the whiteboard spray and cloth. But the board is already clean.

'You don't have to do that,' I say.

He walks over to the whiteboard.

'Are you going to do another course next year?' he asks.

'It will be the same again, Andros,' I say.

'Let me know when it is, OK?'

He sprays the board and wipes it with the cloth.

A few moments later Mooch comes in. He has pale arms, red knuckles and he wears friendship bracelets on both wrists. He's bald on top but has the remainder of his hair in dreadlocks tied back into a ponytail. He takes a drag on his vape.

'We should do a class on UFOs,' Mooch says.

'That's astronomy. This is philosophy,' Andros says.

'Gotta have an open mind though, haven't you? I saw four UFOs last week out my cell window. There was a big one, and then three little ones came out of it. I reckon they must have landed, taken one look at us and realized what horrible violent bastards we was and then gone back home.'

'They must have landed on B-wing then,' Andros says.

'I wish they had. I'd have got them to take me with them,' Mooch says.

Taff walks through the door.

'Oh no! Don't tell me,' Andros says.

Taff looks stricken. He explains how yesterday morning he packed up his belongings, was escorted to reception and waited to be released. His wife waited in the car park. A few hours later, at around midday, he was told there had been a miscommunication between the prison staff regarding his release. The paperwork had not been done. He was taken back onto the landing. He had to move into a new cell, as the one he'd vacated a few hours before had already been taken by someone else. His new cellmate doesn't speak any English.

'I called my solicitor,' Taff says, his voice trembling. 'He says the prison should have released me, but it might take another six weeks. He couldn't give a time.'

'You can get a hundred and fifty quid for each day they keep you in custody that they weren't supposed to,' Mooch says.

'I can't stay here. What if they fuck it up again in six weeks?' Taff says.

'You'd get a big payout then,' Mooch says.

'I called my wife to tell her. She cried for the whole call. She just kept asking when I was coming home. I didn't know what to tell her,' Taff says.

'I had a cellmate in for ten grand of fraud who they kept in two months over by mistake,' Mooch says.

'Am I supposed to tell her that?'

'Fucker got awarded six grand.'

Taff sits down next to Mooch. Andros pats Taff on the shoulder and tells him to make sure he eats today. Mooch says, 'Can't say I'm surprised, Taff. This lot couldn't organize a piss-up in a brewery.'

Andros tuts and says, 'Like you could do a better job of running things. There's 1,300 men in here. This is a major operation.'

'Well, I'd do things very differently if I was in charge,' Mooch says. He takes a drag of his vape. Strawberry-flavoured smoke drifts in the air.

I shut the door and sit at the table with the men. I say, 'In ancient Greece, there was a man called Diogenes, who wanted to live as much in accordance with nature as possible. He slept in a barrel and walked barefoot. People called him Diogenes the Dog. He was proud of that nickname. Once, during a banquet, someone threw a bone at him as a joke. Diogenes lifted his leg and urinated on it.'

'That's gross,' Andros says.

'That's why he did it,' I say. 'He wanted to experience the freedom of doing something shameful without feeling ashamed.'

Mooch laughs a stoner laugh.

I say, 'There is a legend that the ruler of the Greek empire,

Alexander the Great, visited Diogenes while Diogenes was reclining in the sun. Alexander asked if he could do anything for Diogenes. Diogenes replied, "There is something you could do actually."'

'He pissed on him?' Mooch says.

Andros tuts. 'He's Alexander the Great. Not Donald Trump.'

I say, 'Diogenes said to Alexander, "You can move out the way. You're blocking my light."'

'He sounds like my old cellmate,' Andros says. 'When he was in court and the judge asked him to stand, he stood up and turned his back.'

'Diogenes deliberately sought out prosecution. He knew it was a crime to deface the currency, but in his home city of Sinope, he smashed some coins with a hammer. The state exiled him, which he was gleeful about. At the heart of his philosophy was the idea that human nature is at odds with society. He saw exile as freedom.'

'I like this bloke,' Mooch says.

Taff sits slumped, staring at the floor.

I say, 'Diogenes left the gates of Sinope and lived free in the wilderness. Eventually, he came to the gates of Athens. He would have had a choice. He could stay outside and live as he was. Or he could go inside and join society.'

'Whatever you do, don't go in,' Mooch says. 'If he goes in, he's gonna have to live by another man's rules. He'd have to live every day in fear of what they'd do to him if he broke those rules.'

Andros says, 'That fear is there for a reason. It's there so he can be bigger than it. So Diogenes can learn to control himself.'

'It wouldn't be real self-control. It would be society controlling him,' Mooch says.

I tilt my head to try and meet Taff's eye. He glances up, but his facial expression is absent.

Andros says, 'I'm glad that human nature is the opposite of society. Human nature is killing, rape and stealing – just look around this place. You need society. Otherwise, it would be chaos.'

'It's society what makes us bad,' Mooch says. 'I'm in here, OK? I'm a wrong'un. But my half-brother went to private school. He's got a house and two kids. It's society what made him good and me bad.'

Taff looks up. I meet his eye. 'What do you think?' I ask.

'I can't. I can't today,' he says. He looks back at the floor.

In the class, Andros says, 'How does Diogenes know human nature ain't at home in society? He's never seen a human that weren't in society.'

'There has been. Me!' Mooch says.

'You?' Andros says.

'When I was in the seg, that was just me alone for days. I wasn't in society then. It was just pure me. Nothing else. I was just floating in my own consciousness.'

'A prison cell is the most in society you could ever be,' Andros says.

'I didn't have a telly,' Mooch says.

'It don't matter,' Andros says.

'I just lay there feeling the weight of my body against the bed.'

'If you don't have the state and society, then you would have no prisons.'

'I hadn't thought of that,' Mooch says.

He scratches his head.

'What if I went to China and Africa,' he says. 'Once I'd seen loads of different people, I'd know what human nature was.'

'They won't let you into China with a criminal record,' Andros says.

'Yeah,' Mooch says.

Mooch takes a drag of his vape and the smoke billows out from his nostrils. The cloud drifts over towards Taff but Taff doesn't react.

Mooch says, 'You know who Diogenes reminds me of? Me.'

Andros's mouth hangs open. He stares at Mooch, waiting to hear what he's going to say next.

Mooch goes on. 'I never buy anything from the canteen. Canteen day is just like another day for me. I don't give my money to this place. And when the guvs call for association in the yard, I stay in my cell.'

'Why?' I ask.

'Because when I go out, I'm going out for real.'

Mooch tightens his ponytail.

'Big man, I saw you on your mattress eating chocolate biscuits last week,' Andros says.

'But they weren't mine.'

'Bruv, you was holding the packet.'

'It was my birthday. I only had a couple.'

'Mooch, Diogenes don't eat birthday biscuits.'

Mooch laughs whilst inhaling from his vape and goes into a coughing fit. Taff squeezes his eyes shut.

*

I give the men a ten-minute break. Mooch picks up a pen and on the whiteboard he draws a picture of Diogenes pissing on a bone. I smile to myself and think of how Diogenes's outrageousness is the antithesis of Joseph K.'s quivering guilt. Where K. walks a fatalistic path, Diogenes goes in his own direction. At the end of *The Trial*, K. is executed by a knife to the heart and as he's dying he says the words 'Like a dog!', and then the novel closes with the line, 'It was as if the shame would outlive him.' But Diogenes was the dog who had outlived his shame.

The break ends and we get back to the discussion. Fifteen minutes before the end of the lesson, I say, 'Diogenes thought being a philosopher meant you should live outside of conventional life. Another philosopher, Seneca, was adviser to the emperor Nero. He was at the heart of the social order.'

I rest my hand on my thigh. I feel my phone in my pocket.

I lift my hands up and place them flat on the table.

'Weren't Nero the one who used to burn people alive?' Mooch says.

My thighs tense up.

'Tell him to stop blocking your light and he'll go to town on you,' Mooch says. He laughs. His lip rides up to show his top teeth and gums.

For the next fifteen minutes I'm willing the time to pass, as I try not to let the fear show on my face. My mouth is dry. My ears are ringing. An officer in the corridor outside shouts, 'Free flow.' The men file out. Andros wipes the board before he leaves. Taff remains sat in his chair.

I grab my rucksack.

'I hope they let you out, Taff,' I say, my own voice pumping fear into me.

He scoffs. 'They don't give a fuck.'

He gets to his feet and heads back to his cell.

I leave my room and walk down the twos, past a man in a yellow and green escape suit who is carrying plastic plates of food back to his cell. I'm so afraid, my kidneys are aching. A few metres ahead I see an officer patrolling the landing.

The thought flashes into my mind that I have done something bad by bringing my phone into the prison, that I have not just made a mistake. I must have intended to do something criminal. I should go to the officer and tell him.

But I know that is the executioner calling for me.

I walk past the officer to the gate, and I hand in my keys. The electronic security door opens.

I step out of the prison.

I walk away from the gates of the jail. A motorcyclist hurtles past me. I feel a thrill like I were on the bike myself. A grey cat treads along the narrow top of some garden railings. He's pulling off the cheekiest of feats. He's getting away with it in broad daylight.

I feel a lightness that edges on vertigo. In my relief, I'm awash with tenderness. Everything moves me – two gangly teenagers walking home from school together, an old woman shopping stepping onto a bus – everything touches me with its life.

I come to the canal. A narrowboat cruises past me. Inside, an old dog stares at me through the window. I walk along the towpath to where the water meets the river.

Change

> They say, misery is a good school: maybe. But happiness is the best university. It completes the upbringing of the soul, capable for the good and the beautiful.
>
> ALEXANDER PUSHKIN

A week later, I leave prison and go to Hampstead Heath. In the woods, I find a vast, fallen red oak tree. I drop my rucksack on the floor and hoist myself up onto the trunk. I walk along the main body of the tree and climb onto a thick branch that once reached towards the sky but now runs parallel to the ground. I walk along the top of it until a few feet before the wood becomes too thin to take my weight. I sit down. My feet dangle six metres above the earth.

I think, 'What if I have left my phone in prison?' I feel an impulse to check my rucksack to make sure my phone is in there, but I know that is only the executioner calling for me. I focus on the feeling of my weight going into the tree that is supporting me. The dread twists tighter in my stomach.

I gaze into the woods and try to remember that these oaks are hundreds of years old. They existed before me and before this fear. I touch the bark of the tree I'm sitting on. I lightly run my hand over it and I linger at a patch that is smooth.

The dread passes. A tiny euphoria floats up in my chest. The green of the leaves looks one shade brighter.

I feel like I have just done something audacious. I didn't show up to my own execution. It will have to go ahead without me.

At 2 a.m. I wake up feeling ominous. I have the sense that something bad is about to happen to me. I must have done something wrong.

I feel annoyed that this is happening again. I turn on my other side, let out a deep sigh and allow myself to drift back to sleep. I sleep through until the morning. I wake up feeling fresh and rested.

Sometimes it's the anger I feel about the executioner that gives me the determination not to go to him. When my mind is taken by guilt, I always think twice about what I'm doing, what I've done and who I am. It is a state of chronic self-doubt. But when I'm angry, guilt does not stick to me as much; the anger is too physical, too singular for my convoluted thoughts to gain purchase on my mind. One of the most suffocating scenes in *The Trial* is when Joseph K. is on the stand and he loses the capacity to speak. He's given the chance to defend himself, but he can't muster any words. If he'd been able to summon anger then he wouldn't have left it to his prosecutors to tell him who he was.

Over the next few weeks my anxiety is quieter and easier to let go of. I know it will get more intense again at some point, but for now I've decided I'm going to enjoy this reprieve.

My friend Adam has an angular face like me. We also have the same green eyes and thick dark hair as each other. Last February, when I went to visit him in Paris, we discovered that we were each wearing the exact same double-breasted peacoat. When we weren't wearing them, we could tell them apart because mine is a medium and his a large.

At his apartment he showed me an elegant fedora hat he had recently bought for himself.

'I'll take you to the shop where I got it,' he said.

'We shouldn't,' I said.

'Trust me, you feel so sharp in a hat.'

'I'd look like a tribute act version of you,' I said.

We left his apartment, onto the streets of St-Germain. It was a clear blue day. We went to the cinema to see a matinee of an old film set on a clear blue day. Much of our friendship of the last ten years has involved meeting up in exciting cities and going to the cinema. But, for all the ways in which we are similar, Adam and I have radically different chemical compositions. He is passionate about psychoactive drugs. He often eulogizes about the virtues of LSD or MDMA and how they offer access to new paradigms. 'I wanna peer pressure you into it,' he says. I always laugh him off.

Adam's appetite for drugs doesn't seem to come from a need to numb chronic emotional pain but from his commitment to living an expansive and optimistic life. He takes mushrooms, MDMA, DMT or LSD to have adventures in the possibilities of consciousness. I envy him for his freedom.

I sometimes wonder if letting go of my teetotalism could be a way to let go of the pain from which it originated. Holding on to my sobriety keeps me holding on to the past. Next month, I'm going to visit Adam at his flat in Lisbon, a place he moved to specifically because it had decriminalized drugs. When I spoke to him on WhatsApp a few days ago, he told me that the MDMA in the city was of excellent quality.

'I really think I should peer pressure you into it,' he said.

I'm waiting for three more men to arrive before I start the class. I'm worried they've been shipped out to other prisons in the night. Security don't always like people knowing too far in advance when they will be transported, in case they use it as a chance to plan an escape. I ask Campbell, a short man with deep rings around his eyes, if he knows where the other men are.

'David's cellmate has a visit,' Campbell says.

'But does David have a visit?' I ask.

'He's got the cell to himself. He's having a wank.'

I stand at the doorway to look for David and the others. The corridor is empty but for one man banging on the door to the drug rehab wing.

'My name should be on the list!' he shouts through the glass. 'Look again!'

The officer on the other side of the door isn't opening it. It's common knowledge that the drug rehab wing is the best place to score.

'Just let me in. It's to see my friend, I promise,' the man shouts. 'Just for two minutes.'

I close my classroom door. The room is gloomy. It's sunny outside but the windows in here are small and they have thick bars on them. Even in July this prison is like a submarine. I flick the light switch. The fluorescent bulbs come on and the light casts shadows in the depressions beneath Campbell's cheekbones.

I say to the men, 'Imagine a ship called the Ship of

Theseus. Over seven years, the captain replaces every single part of the ship with a new part. Every plank of wood, every nail. The mast and the sail get replaced with new ones too.'

I ask, 'Is it the same ship?'

'Is it still Theseus's ship?' Campbell asks.

'Yes.'

'Then it's still the same ship. If it still belongs to him.'

'Why?'

'When you first come to jail you worry that means you're never gonna be the same person you was before,' Campbell says.

'Does prison make you a different person?' I ask.

'It don't do that to me. My mum still comes and visits me. Not everyone's mum does that in here, but mine does. When she looks at me, she sees the same me she's always seen.'

When I was twenty-one, I was staying in a twin room in a hotel with my brother. In the morning, he went into the en-suite bathroom, shut the door behind him, and rattled the wood in the frame to make sure the lock was secure. Twenty minutes later he was still inside, and I needed the toilet.

I waited outside the door. I heard him sucking air through his teeth.

'I need a piss, Jason,' I said, through the door.

'Just a second.'

I paced up and down the hotel room to take my mind off my bladder. I tried to tiptoe so he couldn't hear me so I didn't make him anxious, slow him down and have to wait longer to piss.

'I love you, Bruv,' he said.

'I know.'

The week following the Ship of Theseus lesson, Campbell isn't here. Another student tells me Campbell has racked up drug debts on the wing that he can't repay. He has been moved to the VP wing for his own protection. Otherwise, he could get his head kicked in or be forced to hold a phone or weapon for a drug dealer. My uncle has told me he knew drug addicts inside who had to pay their debts in sexual favours. Some of the older men who had money knew this and befriended young heroin addicts, offering to lend them cash they knew they wouldn't be able to repay.

I pick up the chair Campbell usually sits in and move it to the back of the room. I ask the men to move closer together to close the circle. They look around awkwardly and stay where they are.

The men here keep themselves to themselves to avoid trouble. This environment isn't conducive to friendship. This prison has 1,300 beds and 33,000 men pass through here in one year. Living here must be like living in an airport. I'm continually having to remind men who sleep on the same landing of each other's names.

David walks into the class. He has pitted skin and is twitchy, his shoulders leaning forward like he's about to pre-emptively attack. He apologizes for missing last week and puts his hand out to shake mine. I pass him the reading from the previous session. He takes a seat and strikes up a conversation with a new student. They are bonding over their shared stomping ground of Catford in south-east London. David says, 'I know Catford well. I go in that pub a lot . . . that's my bookies . . . I'm around there a lot.' He uses the present tense, although he hasn't been around Catford for four years and won't be going back there for at least another three.

I get the class underway, picking up from last week's focus on whether we are the same person we were seven years ago. I say, 'Your skin, hair, the cells in your bone marrow, your attitudes and personality change over time. So, does that mean yo—'

The door opens. An officer in his fifties comes in and walks across the room between the men and me. David crosses his arms. The officer looks through some papers on my desk. His radio is sounding. It is turned up loud. David shakes his head and indignation spreads across his face. The officer picks up a folder and leaves.

'He didn't even say excuse me. Don't we deserve that?' David says.

'I know it's annoying,' I say.

'I ain't annoyed. Screws don't fucking bother me. When I get released, he'll still be coming into the place every day. I'm not the one wasting my life in here. He is.'

I try to refocus him back on the philosophy. 'If everything about you changes, does that mean you change?' I say.

'Fingerprints,' David says. 'Don't matter how much you've changed, you can still get nicked for your fingerprints.'

When my uncle Frank was fifteen, the police caught him and his friend breaking into a shop, stealing jars of gobstoppers and fizzy sweets. The police put Frank in the back seat of their car with an officer sat either side of him. They dropped the shop's cash box in Frank's lap, grabbed his wrists and tried to force his hands onto the box. They wanted his fingerprints on it to make it look as though he had been trying to steal money too. Frank clenched his fists. The two officers tried to prise open his hands, pulling at his thumb and fingers.

Frank kept his fists closed until they arrived at the station, and the officers gave up.

In one of the Victorian prisons I work in, B-wing is the drug rehab wing. There, recovering heroin users get prescribed morphine patches to manage their withdrawal, or they get given lofexidine, a drug that speeds up the clucking and moves them through withdrawal quicker. This is one of the things that makes rehab wings the best place to score. Men will come from other parts of the prison to buy morphine patches, take them back to their cells and chew them to get a buzz. Lofexidine is often sought after too, because if you've not been taking heroin and you take it, it will get you stoned.

Aside from prescription drugs, the B-wing has its fair share of weed and skunk. I've heard men on those wings who were trying to get clean complain about how hard it is to avoid getting passively high when their cellmate is smoking spice. Spice is a synthetic drug that has become popular in prison because it's very hard to detect in a urine test and it comes soaked into sheets of paper. People can easily hide it in books and letters. But it's a violently unpredictable drug. The chemical compound varies from sheet to sheet. Two puffs might get a man high for a few hours. Or it might make them foam at the mouth, claw their eyes out or take their clothes off and run around the exercise yard naked.

I never know what is going to happen when I have men from B-wing in my class. They might be giving it their all to get clean or they could be mildly sleepy or stoned. They might have a fit, vomit, pass out or fall into my arms and cry.

This morning I have a man in my class called Gary who has drooping eyelids and a huge grin on his face. The group are discussing the Ship of Theseus.

'Theseus. He's the one who killed the moo-moo cow,' Gary says.

'The minotaur, yes. Do you think it's the same ship?' I say.

'Dunno. It's up to the cow.'

I turn to the rest of the class. 'What do you guys thi—'

'The same. It's the same,' Gary shouts out.

'Why?' I ask.

'Because.'

He gawps at me. He furrows his brow.

'What was the question again?' he asks.

'If all the parts have been replaced, then is it the same ship?' I say.

'Yes. It is,' he says.

'Why?' I say.

'Cos.'

He closes one eye as if trying to think.

'Wait. What was the question again?' he says.

The next day, I'm in a different prison, having lunch in the staff mess, sitting with a woman called Zodie, who works in healthcare. She tells me that men here are allowed six condoms, but the prison doesn't want people accumulating them because many men use them to secrete drugs in their anuses. Zodie is only allowed to give men a fresh condom if they return a used one to her first.

Adam messaged me last night. He told me he'd been detoxing for a couple of months, tripping out on 'The phenomenology of Andy'. He also said he'd sourced some good quality MDMA ready for my visit. I'm excited, but also worried that I'll get to Lisbon and I won't be able to get the drug ruin I see in prison out of my mind.

After lunch, I'm teaching my class. Among the group are Reg and Yannis. Reg could be forty or sixty. He has a lined face and is missing four front teeth. Yannis is an athletic man who wears his hair tied in a topknot.

I tell the class about *anattā*, the Buddhist idea that there is no fixed self through time. We are changing from minute to minute. Our belief in a self is an ego attachment, a delusion and a cause of suffering. According to Buddhism, none of us are ever the same person we were yesterday.

Reg writes 'anattā' on the heel of his hand. He's on remand and says he'll bring up anattā at his hearing when they ask him if he was still a danger to society.

Yannis says, 'But you'll be changing from minute to minute. What if you change into a criminal again?'

'Well, I'll stop being a Buddhist once I get out,' Reg says.

Yannis laughs. 'You already sound enlightened.'

Reg says, 'Every time you come back to prison, they issue you with the same number what you had for your last sentence. Don't matter if you're out for ten days or ten years; you get the same number.'

'Prison stays with you even when you get out,' Yannis says. 'Some things you remember even if you don't want to. It's like when you've looked into the sun and you look away and you can't help but see that spot in your vision.'

'So, are you the same person?' I ask.

Yannis says, 'The only thing that matters is how you become different. Are you different because you've transformed, or because you've been changed?'

'What's the difference?' Reg says, his words wet-sounding from the gap in his teeth.

Yannis says, 'When a man has transformed, he's built himself. When he's been changed, he's been destroyed. Some people come into prison and they get changed by it. They get fat. They don't talk to anyone. Get addicted to drugs they didn't even try until they came here. But you can transform in here too if you stay focused.'

'If someone transforms, are they the same person?' I ask.

'You transform whilst you're being changed. Prison makes you stronger and weaker at the same time.'

The officers call free flow. Twenty minutes later, in the staffroom, the teachers are talking about Ted, one of my students. Ted is a little under five feet tall and is the gobbiest person I have ever encountered in prison. On the landing, he walks up to the henchest man he can find and says, 'Get out of the fucking road, I've got places to be,' or, 'Stop blocking the doorway, you're making the place look untidy.' Yet, no harm ever seems to come to him. The men just look down at him, bemused and step out of the way. If they argued back or squared up to him it would somehow be more humiliating for them than it would be for Ted.

One of the teachers, Dana, tells me that last year in court Ted put his fingers in his ears whilst the judge was giving him his sentence. I'm sceptical. Those kinds of stories are often apocryphal, inflated or borrowed from someone else on the landing.

'Did he tell you that?' I ask her.

'Google him if you don't believe me,' she says.

In the evening, on my phone, I type Ted's name into my browser, followed by the word 'jailed'. I hit enter. An article comes up. It confirms that Ted did indeed put his fingers in his ears whilst the judge was sentencing him.

The article has an image of Ted's mugshot taken on the day of his arrest. He looks like he has just woken up. I laugh. The photo captures nothing of the cocky man I know. It seems incongruent that this should be the image used to represent him.

I wonder about my other students. How big is the gap between the image I have of them and public story about who they are? I type in Yannis's name and hit enter. An article with CCTV footage comes up. In broad daylight, Yannis is running away from the scene of his crime to the end of the road and out of shot. His hoodie looks baggy on his drug-eaten body. The frame cuts to another CCTV camera picking him up on the next street. He runs down the road and out of the frame again. The screen cuts to another camera picking him up. After two and a half minutes, Yannis is still running, as the video fades to black.

I close my laptop, wondering if I have committed some kind of betrayal. As a teacher, I'm supposed to care more about what Yannis's future could be rather than what he has done in the past.

A few days later, on the landing, I see Yannis sitting on a plastic chair that's bolted to the floor. We chat. Maybe he can tell from the new inflection in my voice, but he makes a point of telling me how things were in his life in the years leading to his arrest. He tells me that his mental health was crazy and he owed thousands of pounds to drug dealers. It is as if he can tell I know something about him that I didn't know the last time we spoke.

A few hours later, I leave the prison and go to the fallen tree. A boy, around age nine, is crouched down, hiding in the tangle of horizontal branches. Another boy sneaks up to the tree. He puts his arm through the branches and tags the boy crouching there on the head. He turns and runs away. The boy climbs out from the branches and chases the child who has just tagged him. I stand and watch them disappear into the woods.

I lean against the tree, take out my phone and delete the articles about Ted and Yannis from my history.

The following evening, I'm eating damp chips from a cardboard tray in a fast food place in Lisbon with Adam. We catch up on books we've read and films we've seen. Adam finishes his hot dog, goes to the counter and comes back with another one. I push the tray of half-eaten chips away from me and say 'Have your ever read Primo Levi's essay *Shame*?' Adam shakes his head and chomps into his hot dog.

I fill him in on it. 'He lost the world,' I say. 'When I read him I still try and look for the ways he could have got it back.'

'Huh. Last year my friend Benjamin invited me around to his for Passover,' Adam says, one side of his mouth full of food. 'When he dished up, before we ate, he told us how it was important to savour the food because those who were in the camps weren't able to.'

I grimace. 'How were you supposed to do that when you're thinking of people in Auschwitz?'

'That's kinda what makes the meal special. You're supposed to enjoy it on their behalf.'

I look down at my chips. If I tried to savour that meal, I wouldn't be able to not feel like I was being obnoxious.

'Are you gonna finish those?' Adam says, pointing at my chips.

'You have them,' I say.

A few minutes later, two of Adam's friends join us. Adam says that now is the optimum time to go to his favourite club. 'Let's get there whilst it's nice and mellow. Come 1 a.m., it'll be nothing short of a bacchanalia.' He takes four pale green pills out of his pocket. He and his two mates take one. 'I'll take mine when we get there,' I say.

An hour later, we're sat facing an oval-shaped swimming pool on the top floor of the club. There are beds around the edge of the room. On one of them, two men and two women are cuddling together. Silk fabric is draped from the ceiling above them. Dim orange light comes from the Moroccan-style hanging lamps. The DJ is playing a techno track with a slow hypnotic beat.

Adam's pupils are dilated and he has an enormous grin on his face. He takes a pill out of his pocket and offers it to me.

'I feel too guilty,' I say.

'This will make you feel pure innocence,' he says.

'I'm gonna swim,' I say to Adam. I take my shoes and socks off.

'I'll keep it safe for you,' Adam says and puts the pill back in his jeans pocket.

I walk over to the pool, take off my jeans and T-shirt and climb down into the water. I hold my breath, dip my head under the surface and dive down to the bottom. The sound of the music is blunted through the water. I reach my hands out in front of me and swim.

I come up for air and Adam is stood at the side of the pool.

'You were swimming underwater, Andy,' he says exuberantly. 'Then you came back up,' he says exuberantly.

I see the two men and two women on the bed. They are playing with each other's hair. One of the men is squeezing his eyes shut in pleasure.

I put my head under the water and dive back down to the bottom.

A few weeks later, I'm in a new prison, and in the morning, I'm told I'll be working today on F-wing – the drug rehab wing. I've heard that this rehab wing is genuinely more therapeutic than the ones like B-wing that Gary was on. Men have to prove they are clean to get on it, and I've met men who have been kicked off the wing who talk about it nostalgically. I've also spoken to people who left therapeutic groups in prison by choice because they found it traumatic listening to other people talk about their gruesome crimes, or they felt coerced into talking for fear they'd be labelled 'Defiant' in their file. Many people in prison might benefit from therapy, but therapy under incarceration is an extremely complicated issue.

At 2 p.m. I walk to F-wing. I don't have the special key for this door. I press the buzzer and wait to be let in. Through the window, I see tattered plastic bags caught in the rings of razor wire on the fence.

An officer opens the door, searches me and lets me

through. Apparently, F-wing is a special secure area. The officer tells me that this wing was set up as a prison within a prison in the eighties and nineties to hold members of the IRA and people who might try and escape. But today, F-wing's strict security isn't to stop anyone getting out, it's to stop drugs from getting in. Corrupt staff are one of the main ways drugs get into prison. That's why I had to be searched. Men on this wing still have to take urine tests every few days. Anyone who tests positive is sent back to the other wings and not allowed to return for a minimum of three months.

I step onto the wing and hear the sound of a guitar. A man is reclining in a chair playing arpeggios. He has colour in his cheeks. His hair is glossy. He picks the strings of his guitar and hums a melody.

He puts his guitar down and introduces himself as Aiden. He walks me towards my classroom. Painted on the wall are the words, 'Grant me the serenity to accept the things I cannot change, courage to change the things I can, and wisdom to know the difference.' A man in flip-flops approaches me and asks what I'm here for. I tell him and he wants to know more about philosophy. I'm not used to encountering curiosity so openly on the landing.

Aiden and I get to the classroom. We set out six chairs. A man with bright eyes and a scar three inches long across his cheek comes in. His name is Tyrese. He and Aiden give each other a hug, slapping each other on the back. They sit next to each other. Their knees are less than an inch apart from one another's.

Three other men come in and take a seat. I get the lesson underway. We discuss if the Ship of Theseus is the same ship it was and the question of whether people are the same individual over time too.

'When I look at a photo of me from when I was using, I don't say, "That is me," I say, "That was me,"' Aiden says.

'So you're a different person, you think?' Tyrese says.

'I can't say that yet. That's only a photo. It only shows the outside,' Aiden says.

'Right now, I'm changing how I think and how I act,' Tyrese says. 'I wake up in the mornings and I've got energy. For years I found the food a chore, but now I want to eat all the time.'

'But that don't make you a different person. Just because you're a morning person now don't mean you can't still go and smash someone's face in tomorrow,' Aiden says.

'True. I used to want people to look at me and see someone with the aura of a killer. But now, I hope that one day the people I've let down might be able to trust me again.'

'But how do you do that? How do you prove to people you've become a different person?' Aiden says.

'It's like the ship. The ship is only different once all the parts have been repaired. We've only changed the first bit of ourselves in here. We have to keep going,' Tyrese says.

'People used to look at me and see a thug,' Aiden says. 'My attitude was, "If you call me a thug, then I'll show you a thug!" I wanted to be worse than the worst thing people thought about me. But that wasn't who I really was. I feel like I've only just started to learn who I am since I've come here.'

'You just have to keep going. Keep repairing,' Tyrese says.

★

Twenty minutes later, an officer comes in, leans against the wall and listens. The men carry on talking. Aiden nods at the officer and the officer nods back. The atmosphere is much softer here than it is in the main prison. The men look at ease being open with each other. I haven't had to break up rows from where a disagreement has turned nasty. There are still bars on the windows and officers with cell keys on their belt, but there is an optimism in the room that I rarely feel with a group in prison.

Thirty seconds from the end of class, I ask the men, 'So, is it the same ship?'

'It will become a different ship once you replace all the parts,' Tyrese says.

'I don't know yet what it is,' Aiden says.

The men file out to get ready for their evening group-therapy session. Aiden gives me a warm handshake, looks into my eyes and says, 'Thank you.' He leaves, and I close the door behind him.

I sit and watch the light change outside the window. The central building of the prison looks flat against the late afternoon sky.

I pack up my things, go out onto the landing and wait for the guard to unlock the security door. Through an open cell, I see Aiden, topless and bent over his sink. Tyrese stands to the side of him, shaving the back of Aiden's neck. Aiden rests his forearms on the sink. His shoulder blades stick out towards the ceiling. Tyrese blows on Aiden's neck to get rid of the shavings.

Three weeks later, I'm with Adam and some other friends, in the same club we were in before. A good-looking couple are making out in the middle of the pool. Adam tells me he has an MDMA pill for me.

'I've been keeping it safe for you,' he says,

'I'll take half of it,' I say.

'Andy, you're in such a beautiful setting. You're with friends. It would be a great shame if you under-dosed.'

I take the pill, put it in my mouth and swallow.

Four days later, I'm still in a splendid afterglow. Adam and I are walking down the street in Lisbon and an oncoming stranger bumps into my shoulder. It's the most wonderful surprise. We stop at a cafe and I ask for two colas. The waiter comes and puts my drink on the table. The circular rim of the bottle is astonishing to me.

I show it to Adam.

'Look. We are so lucky to have the universe,' I say.

'We are,' he says.

We burst out laughing at one another.

MDMA temporarily drowned out the voice in my head that told me happiness was obnoxious. It allowed me to experience uncensored joy. Although the chemical high has faded, I'm still amazed by ordinary sensations. A week later, I fly back to London. On Monday morning, I go into prison. The fluorescent strip lights are mesmeric. I push open an iron bar door. The metal feels so smooth. Walking down the landing, I bump into Yannis.

'Did you have a good weekend?' I say. I usually make a point to avoid asking people inside this question, but I'm less able to filter my words than I was. But Yannis tells me that he did have a good weekend. On Friday he received a letter from a friend he hadn't seen for a few years. Yannis was delighted to have six pages of somebody else's news. He read the letter several times over the weekend, sometimes pausing between sentences so that he could live a little longer in the scenes being described. He is looking forward to responding, but he doesn't want to write a reply right away. He wants to enjoy the excitement of having a letter to write back for a few days. At night, when the officers call lights out, he'll lie on his bed and think of the questions he's going to ask his friend.

At five o'clock, I leave the prison and go and sit with my friend Johnny in his garden. We talk for a couple of hours and notice the light is starting to change. Johnny makes a small bonfire out of a pile of branches. I'm happy that we will get to be together here a little longer. I think of Yannis and how excited he was about sending a letter to his friend. Somehow that thought makes being here with Johnny all the more special.

The sun goes down completely. Johnny stands up, breaks a long branch in half and puts it on the fire. He sits back down next to me and I feel joy on Yannis's behalf.

I thought about my brother whilst I was high. I didn't think of him injecting between his toes or getting stabbed over a drug debt. I thought of the love he shares with his kids and that he has a place where he feels at home. I was happy for him. For the first time since I was a child, I experienced what it was like to see him without pity.

The weekend after returning from Lisbon, I'm in McDonald's with my brother. We use the self-service counter to browse what we want. The touch screen display is so sleek and beautiful. We order two chocolate milkshakes, collect our ticket and wait at the counter for our number to be called out.

'I got high recently,' I tell him.

'Are you joking?' he says.

'I took some MDMA,' I say.

'Really?'

'Really.'

He furrows his brow.

'Are you OK?' I ask.

'I'm relieved,' he murmurs.

The worker behind the counter calls out our number. Jason and I collect our milkshakes. We find two stools next to each other facing the window and we sit down.

'I thought I'd damaged you forever,' he says.

'Jason, I had so much fun.'

Stories

> No need of a story, a story is not compulsory,
> just a life, that's the mistake I made, one of the
> mistakes, to have wanted a story for myself,
> whereas life alone is enough.
>
> SAMUEL BECKETT

Four years ago, shortly after I'd started working in prisons, I was at my nan's on a Sunday afternoon. The TV was playing the *EastEnders* omnibus. Frank was sat on the arm of the sofa opposite me, rolling a cigarette.

'There was a VCR shop we burgled about four times,' he said.

I'd heard this story from him several times before, but I let him go on. He told the same stories about prison over and over. Again and again, I listened to them, like songs I'd long since learnt all the words to. I listened for the crackle of glee in his voice and the cadence of his punchlines. The story of my relationship with my uncle was that he told me stories. Although it so often felt like there was a wall between us, I liked to think that when he was telling me a story, an imaginary thread connected us. It was like he was Theseus, inside the labyrinth, holding one end of the thread, and I was Ariadne, outside, holding the other end.

He carried on. 'Each time me and Vinnie burgled it we did exactly the same thing. It was a doddle. We went in through the roof, inside there was a plaster floor with all wooden beams on top of it. I knelt on a beam and poked my finger through the plaster. I kept picking at the hole, making it bigger.'

I knew that next, he would tell me about the copper wires embedded in the plaster.

'There was copper wires in the plaster, about three inches apart. If you snap them it sets off the alarm. So I picked a hole about three metres big, wide enough for the wires to hang slack. Then I parted them.'

He mimed the gesture of parting the wires, spearing his hands downwards and gently stroking them apart.

'Wow,' I said, as if hearing this story for the first time.

On the wall outside my classroom is a picture, drawn by a student in the art class, of a skeleton reading a book. Every bone has been drawn in detail. Last week the speech bubble coming from the skeleton's mouth read, 'It's never to late to start education,' but I see that someone has since tried to correct it. Now it says, 'It's never toolate to start education.'

I lean against the wall in the corridor, waiting for morning free flow to start. Diagonally opposite me is a display board listing the companies open to employing ex-prisoners. Officer Collins, a Mancunian woman who is currently studying for a diploma in life-coaching, is sticking LGBT posters to the board. One includes a photo of a trans man and some text where he describes his experience.

Collins can't reach high enough up the wall to mount the laminated photo of a Pride flag in her hand. She asks me to help and points to where she wants me to stick it, about a foot from the ceiling.

'Last month I put a Pride flag low down and it went missing,' she says.

'Not surprised. This place is so homophobic.'

'It wasn't that. We found the missing flag in someone's cell, on the wall.'

'That was brave of him, to display it like that,' I say.

'He was an old-age pensioner. He didn't know what a Pride flag was. He just liked the colours and wanted to brighten up his cell.'

I stand on tiptoes and stick the image to the wall. An officer shouts, 'Free flow!' I go and stand outside my classroom. There are new rules that students must line up in the corridor until free flow has finished like you would in a Victorian boarding school.

Tommy is the first man to arrive. He has a substantial build, as if his body is made from timber, and he walks with a slight sway but steadily. Last month, he told me that he's been inside for ten years and isn't due to be released for another decade. 'But it makes the world a better place,' he said. 'If me being punished means that in the future less people will do what I did, then I have to accept it.' Deep down, I knew his story didn't hold; prison is a lousy deterrent, especially for the type of crime he'd committed. But I didn't want to say that to him; I didn't even want to think it to myself. I found his equanimity beautiful. I wanted it to last a little bit longer.

Tommy carries a clear A3-sized folder in his hand. He rediscovered his talent for art in his late twenties, when he began his sentence. A few weeks ago, he showed me his work. There were a dozen drawings of his own hands, a still life of some teabags from his canteen and a line drawing of the barbed wire he can see from his cell window. I asked him if he wanted to do portraits. 'Lockdowns always scupper portraits,' he said. 'Easier to draw stuff that doesn't depend on other people.'

In the corridor, I ask Tommy what he's working on at the moment. He takes out an A4 piece from his folder and hands it to me. It is a painting of tropical birds and flowers. A toucan with a long yellow beak. A red hibiscus. Some parakeets and frangipani are sketched in but not yet painted.

'I did it from an advert in the paper for holidays in Brazil,' Tommy says.

An officer escorts an old man down the corridor. The officer has rosy cheeks, big ears and blond hairs above his top lip. He looks about nineteen or twenty. The old man has a hearing aid behind one of his thick ears and a neat comb-over across the top of his scalp. The prison service has been desperate to recruit new staff in recent years and the minimum age to become a prison officer is eighteen. Meanwhile, convictions for historic crimes and longer sentences has meant there are more pensioners in prison than ever.

The two exit the corridor. It's most likely they are going to healthcare.

Over the next few minutes, the corridor is filling up. A man shoulders into me. I step back closer to the wall. Tommy puts the painting back in his folder to protect it. A student called Lafferty arrives. He's about sixty, has a thick Belfast accent and wears a red woolly hat that's pulled so tightly onto his head that it covers his eyebrows.

Lafferty points at Tommy's folder and tells us that he's covered his cell walls in pictures of sports cars he's cut out from magazines. 'My cell looks like a millionaire's garage,' he says.

'Love it, mate,' Tommy says.

'What did you say?' Lafferty says.

'Your cell sounds sweet, mate, that's all,' Tommy says.

'You called me mate. Are you a homo?' Lafferty says.

Me and Tommy look at each other, confused.

'Watch!' Lafferty says, announcing that he's about to hold forth. 'In the animal kingdom, do you know what "mate" means? It means fucking. When a homo says mate to you, they're trying to fuck you.'

I try not to laugh. 'What do you call your cellmate then, Lafferty?' I ask.

'My bunkie,' he says. He turns and takes a few steps down the corridor to a group of teenagers standing in front of the display board.

'He doth protest too much, methinks,' Tommy says to me.

'How is "bunkie" any less gay than "mate"?'

Lafferty high-fives each one of the five teenagers in turn. 'Watch,' Lafferty says and launches into a monologue. 'Three years is an easy thing. Let me tell you about the time I did seven and a half years. I did every day of it.' The teenagers listen, their mouths hanging open. Lafferty's nickname in prison is the Pied Piper. All the children want to follow him.

'You should always hit a man back,' Lafferty says to the boys. He doesn't seem to realize that he's giving his lecture under the Pride flag high up on the wall. His woolly hat must be covering the top part of his vision.

★

More men cram into the corridor. Tommy has to shout so I can hear him. I can smell the morning breath of the man to my side. In front of me, a tall bald man with a pinched roll of flesh at the back of his head steps backwards and I hold him off by pressing my forearm against his lower back. I feel the warm sweat through his T-shirt.

An officer shouts, 'End of free flow.' I unlock my classroom, and Lafferty and Tommy go inside. The corridor clears but for three teenagers. Two of them are beatboxing for the third one, who is rapping. I can only make out some of the words, but he seems to be talking about racism in the justice system.

An officer walking the corridor says, 'Free flow is over, gentlemen. Inside, please.'

The boys keep rapping. There is a line about how Africans weren't always drug dealers but were once kings and queens.

'Classrooms or cells. Your choice!' the officer shouts.

One of the beatboxers is my student, G. He fist bumps his two friends and walks over to me. He has puppy-fat cheeks and both his arms are inked with tattoos from knuckle to bicep.

'What are your tattoos of?' I ask him.

'One arm is life. The other is death,' G says.

On his left arm, he has a tree and a pregnant woman and a scroll with curly writing on. On his right arm, he has a skull in a swirling vortex and a scroll again.

'What are the scrolls of?' I say.

'Just life and death. That's what the man in the shop said. I was gonna get life on one arm, death on the other and then loads of tattoos on my chest of stuff in between. But then I came to jail.'

We step inside the class together. I shut the door behind me.

A few minutes later, in my classroom, Tommy and G sit opposite each other. Outside they were both roadmen, only Tommy is twenty years further into that life than G. Tommy wears bootcut jeans, where G wears tracksuit bottoms that sit halfway down his ass, but they've both been through the same poverty, adversity and violence. Lafferty sits between them, his legs spread wide apart. I pull up a chair and sit in front of the three men. I give each a printout of an image of *David with the Head of Goliath*, by Caravaggio. It shows the boy David holding the decapitated head of the giant Goliath by the hair. The figures are standing in darkness. David's face is melancholic. Goliath's eyes are still bright with pain.

'David was smart,' Lafferty says. He taps the side of his head.

'He doesn't look happy considering he's just killed the giant,' Tommy says.

I say, 'There are three interesting things about this painting. Firstly, it's a self-portrait. The decapitated giant has the face of Caravaggio. Secondly, it might be a double self-portrait. The face of David strongly resembles a portrait of the young Caravaggio. Caravaggio might be showing us a picture of his younger self slaying his older self.'

'Oh no. Suicide watch,' G says.

'Thirdly, Caravaggio hoped this painting would redeem him.'

'What did he do?' G asks.

'I need to give you some background before I get to that,' I say. 'Caravaggio was born during the plague, and by the time he was six years old, all the men in his life had died. As an adult, Caravaggio enjoyed the night. He loved gambling, women, drink and frequently had duels with other men.'

'Caravaggio was a gangster,' says G.

'He died young, didn't he?' Tommy says.

'Once, a priest offered to sprinkle holy water on Caravaggio to cleanse him of his mortal sins,' I say. 'Caravaggio replied, "That won't help. All of my sins are cardinal sins."'

'What does that mean?' G says.

'It means he made his own rules, like a man,' Lafferty says.

'Or he didn't believe he could be saved,' Tommy says.

G looks at Lafferty and then at Tommy.

'He was often arrested and thrown in a cell for fighting. But his talent meant he had so many friends in high places that he could go free the next day. Victims dropped the charges, or witnesses suddenly got amnesia. But at thirty-five, Caravaggio had a beef with a man called Ranuccio Tomassoni over a woman or a gambling debt and the two had a duel. Caravaggio slashed an artery in Tomassoni's thigh and he bled to death. The Pope heard of this and declared that Caravaggio must be punished this time. He put a bounty on Caravaggio's head. Caravaggio fled to Naples and went into hiding.'

G throws his arms up in the air. 'Tomassoni fucked his girl. What was Caravaggio supposed to do, just sit there and take it? If he'd walked away, everyone would think he was a pussy.'

I hold up the image of *David with the Head of Goliath*. 'That's when Caravaggio painted this picture.'

I point to the sword resting across David's thigh. The letters "H-AS OS" are inscribed on the blade.

'"H-AS OS" stands for "humility kills pride",' I say.

'Caravaggio sent the painting to Scipione Borghese, the chief administrator for justice in Rome. He sent it as a plea for clemency.'

'How much was the painting worth?' Lafferty says. 'Everything in the world works by money. If that picture is worth a lot of money, Caravaggio can buy his life back from Borghese. It's as simple as that.'

I ask, 'What should Borghese say?'

Tommy says, 'I look at the painting and I think Caravaggio is saying to Borghese, "If you wanna try and hurt me then good luck. You can't hurt me any more than I've hurt myself. I'm way past fearing you."'

'I'd give Caravaggio a second chance,' G says.

Tommy carries on. 'Caravaggio's boasting about how self-destructive he is. The picture is him saying, "This is who I have always been and who I will always be. Take me back and I'll be just the same."'

'But the faces look real sad. He can't stop thinking about what he's done,' G says.

Tommy says, 'If you pardon him, then you start a feedback mechanism. Being a bad boy is part of his art. He knows he's a good artist and that lets him get away with it. If Rome pardons him after this, Caravaggio is gonna know that he can take the piss as much as he likes.'

'He's saying he's sorry, though,' G says.

'He's too arrogant to know how to apologize,' Tommy says.

G tuts and says, 'Do you know what the judge told me? "You need to stop being so smart." He didn't like that I was talking back to him.'

'The painting is too composed. The giant and the boy. The light and the dark. He's relying on his talent instead of facing the remorse,' Tommy says.

'Next time I'm in court, I'm just gonna stand there and pretend I'm too much of an idiot to know what's happening. I bet you they give me an easier sentence.'

'There's no way I'd let him back into Rome,' Tommy says.

A moment later, the door opens. An officer with a bright sunburnt face steps into the room. He says, 'There was a large hardback dictionary on that back table in this room. Whoever took it needs to put it back.'

'It couldn't have been me, guv, I've already got a very well-endowed vocabulary,' says G, his hand down his tracksuit bottoms.

'Was it you that took it?' the officer says to G.

'If I wanted to rob you, I'd properly rob you. I wouldn't do it over a pissy dictionary,' G says.

'It needs to be returned,' the officer says, looking at each man in turn.

'Why you asking me?' Tommy says, 'I've got another ten to do. That dictionary ain't long enough for me to bother stealing.'

The officer leaves, closing the door behind him.

The thin paper of a dictionary makes for decent cigarette paper in prison, especially since Rizlas have officially become contraband. Someone could also use the pages of a dictionary to cover the gap between their cell door and the door frame, so smoke won't seep out of their cells onto the landing when they are smoking, which would allow the officers to catch them. If someone hollowed out a strip in the pages of the dictionary, they could hide a shank inside. Or they could rip off the hardback cover, tuck it into their trousers and have it underneath their T-shirt, to act as armour to protect them from shanks. But jailcraft aside, the dictionary is sought after in prison because people who aren't sure how to spell want to get it right when they draft a legal letter or write to their loved ones.

Tommy says, 'I used to have a cellmate who tried to stop the cockroaches from coming in by scrunching up the pages of a dictionary and using them to plug the holes in our cell wall. Sadly, the cockroaches didn't have as much respect for the English language as he'd hoped. They ate their way through the paper, and he woke up with them crawling over his feet in the middle of the night.'

'I bet it was an officer who nicked the dictionary,' Lafferty says. 'They are worth about twenty-five quid brand new. They've robbed it and are blaming it on us.'

G tilts his head to look at the art folder leaning against Tommy's chair. 'Did you draw those?' G asks. Tommy hands G his folder, passing it in front of Lafferty.

Tommy says, 'I don't believe Caravaggio really wanted to go back to Rome. I think he thrives on being on the run. The buzz of it feeds his art. It's part of the organized chaos he creates in his life to be creative.'

G opens the folder, takes out a few sheets of paper and looks at them.

Tommy says, 'I think Caravaggio doesn't want to be arrogant, but he can't help it. It keeps coming through. It says humility kills pride on the sword, but that's what he wants to be happening, not what has actually happened.'

G pulls out the pictures of the Brazilian birds and flowers. 'This is so cool,' he says.

Tommy says, 'He didn't really care if he had humility or pride. He cared more about art than he did about real life. I guess because he'd seen so much death as a kid. He disappeared into his painting.'

'I want this as my next tattoo,' G says.

A moment later, I ask Lafferty, 'What do you think Borghese should say?'

'He should tell Caravaggio to come back and fight him like a man,' Lafferty says.

The officer looks through the glass of the classroom door. G blows him a kiss.

'Did they let him back into Rome?' Tommy asks me.

'In the end, Borghese wanted to pardon Caravaggio, but he couldn't get enough political support,' I say. 'Caravaggio lived on the run for a few years, briefly joining the Knights of Malta, before getting kicked out for fighting. When he was thirty-eight, the new administration in Rome pardoned him, but two days later, before he could return, he died on the beach in Naples. The cause of his death is unknown. He may have been attacked by an enemy, or fugitive life may have taken its toll on his body. He was thrown into an unmarked grave.'

'Borghese is a dick,' G says. 'He could have saved Caravaggio.'

'It's not Borghese's job to look after a murderer,' Tommy says.

'Caravaggio was born into all that death, and now he's dead too. They never gave a fuck about him,' G says.

'Caravaggio blew it,' Tommy says.

The following Sunday, I'm at my nan's. The TV is playing the *EastEnders* omnibus. I tell Nan I'm not hungry, but she sets out a plate of four custard slices on the coffee table. My uncle sits on the arm of the sofa, slurping a mug of tea. He tells me about the time the police tried to prise his fists open so they could get his fingerprints on a cash box. When he laughed so hard in court, the judge thought he was crying and gave him an easier sentence. When he was a teenager and dug holes eight feet deep, only for the guards to tell him to fill them back in at the end of the day. I listen and eat three custard slices one after the other. I can feel a burning in my stomach from the sugar.

Frank and I can no longer pass as Theseus and Ariadne. We have become trapped inside a narrative loop together. We are stuck in the story of him telling me stories.

My nan asks me if I want to finish the last custard slice. I say no thank you and she goes to the kitchen, brings back a plate of chocolate eclairs and puts it on the coffee table.

'This one time, me, Vinnie and Carl was burgling this warehouse up north,' Frank says. 'Vinnie was outside in the van. He couldn't help shifting the gear cos of his dodgy hip. I was carrying a load of skiing jackets out to the van when we saw this police car coming towards us.'

Frank sets his tea down on the coffee table and rubs his hands together.

'Me and Carl jumped into the van. Vinnie put his foot down and he rams the police car. I said, "Fuck, let's go."'

This is the story where they are pensioners. I pick up a chocolate eclair and put it on my plate.

'The police chased us down the motorway. Where we've rammed them, they think we're young and game and up for it. At each junction, another car came on. There was about fourteen of them chasing us in the end. It was fucking electric. I've got the CCTV tape of it upstairs. We should watch it. Anyway, after about fifty miles we run out of petrol. I said, "Fuck it. We're nicked. Let's pull over."'

I swallow a mouthful of eclair. I feel my stomach burning again.

'I remember you telling me this one,' I say.

'A big black truck pulled up behind us,' he says. 'About six police get out with riot shields and pepper spray. They were wearing helmets and stab-proof vests. They surrounded the van.'

I suck my teeth to try and get the sugar off them. I take another mouthful.

'We got out of the van with our hands in the air. The police have raised their shields. They shone a torch at us. Vinnie covered his eyes from the light. Four coppers grabbed him and cuffed him. I said, "Be careful with him, he's not well."'

I put my plate back on the coffee table. I try not to touch my clothes with my sticky fingers.

'The coppers lowered their shields. One of them said to another one, "Sarge, they're pensioners!"'

'Yeah. I need to wash my hands,' I say.

The next morning at work, I step into the library to use the photocopier and see five men sat around a table in church-like silence. One of my ex-students is there, Vince. He's about six foot five and has thick, muscular arms. He's turning through the pages of a copy of *The Very Hungry Caterpillar*. The other men around the table are reading books like *The Ugly Duckling* and *Aliens love Underpants*.

Some of these men are in custody eighty or ninety miles from their families, and so the price of train and taxi fares makes it hard for relatives to visit regularly. This morning the men will record themselves reading a children's book. The recording will be burnt onto a CD and sent to their children.

I go over to the table and fist bump Vince. I ask him how he is, and he tells me that looking forward to today has allowed him to stay positive for the last two months.

'It's my voice,' he says. 'It makes me feel so much better, knowing that my little girl can hear my voice whenever she wants. The only other time she gets to hear me is when I call her. But then she can hear the banging and screaming of the wing in the background. This one time, I called her up and could hear in the background she was listening to a CD of me reading to her. I choked up. I had to hang up and call her back ten minutes later once I'd sorted myself out.'

'What are you going to read her this time?' I ask.

'I always think I'm gonna read her something new that she ain't heard before, but I always end up reading her one of the books that she knows from me reading it to her from before I went to jail.'

One of the men at the table, Musab, says to me, 'I didn't know about any of these books before I came to prison.' He holds up a copy of *Little Miss Sunshine*. 'This one is actually really good, you know.'

Another man at the table flicks through a book. His eyes

are hard and wet. 'It's moments like this that you realize what you've done,' he says.

I once told a prisoner that my dad had been inside. He looked down at the floor so he didn't have to look at me and think of his son.

I say goodbye to Vince, go into the back room and use the photocopier. I turn around to get more paper, but I'm halted as my key chain gets caught on a door handle. I unhook it. The chain jangles as it drops back to my side.

Musab and a librarian in a corduroy jacket come into the room and sit down. The librarian sets up a recording device. He waits for the copying machine to finish printing. He presses record on his device.

'Say your name and prison number into the microphone, please,' the librarian says.

'Musab Abdulwehab. Prison number P44IX41. I'm going to be— Wait, will my little girl hear my prison number?'

'No. It's just for our records. We'll edit your number out before we send it to her,' the librarian says.

'My name is Musab Abdulwehab. Prison number P44IX41. I'm going to be reading *Little Miss Sunshine*. Hello, darling – this is Daddy.'

Musab reads the story into the microphone. I keep still so the recording doesn't have the sound of my key chain jangling in the background.

Thirty minutes later, in the classroom. Tommy sits with his art folder on the table in front of him. He got up at five this morning so he could meditate. He says that's the only time the wing is quiet enough for him to properly concentrate. G sits opposite, with his head resting on the table.

'Let's start,' I say.

G sits up and stretches.

'I told the screw I wanted to stay in bed. This place is bullshit. When I get out of here, I'm gonna sleep as much as I like,' he says.

I get the lesson underway. I say, 'Caravaggio's pardon came too late. But another artist, Dostoyevsky, got his just in time. Dostoyevsky was sentenced to death for speaking out against the state. He was marched to a square in Saint Petersburg, stood against a wall and blindfolded. A firing squad pointed their guns at him. He heard them cocking their rifles.'

G opens his mouth and yawns.

I say, 'Dostoyevsky stood there waiting to die when a state messenger arrived on horseback. He explained that the Tsar had decided to take mercy on Dostoyevsky. He would now only have to do six years of hard labour in the penal colony. The firing squad lowered their rifles. Dostoyevsky's blindfold was removed.'

G rubs his eyes.

I say, 'Later in his life, Dostoyevsky wrote a novel called *The Idiot*, which included a character named Prince Myshkin, who was spared before a firing squad. After Myshkin's reprieve, he believes absolutely in forgiveness. Whenever someone harms or insults him, he instantly lets it go. Another of Dostoyevsky's books, *Crime and Punishment*, tells the story of Raskolnikov, a man who kills two people to see if he can live out his superman fantasies of living beyond the boundaries of good and evil. But afterwards, Raskolnikov is tormented by his conscience. He's dogged by nightmares.'

'That's good, right? That means you're not a psychopath

if you have nightmares about the stuff you've done, isn't it?' G says.

'In the end, he turns himself in to the police so he can start his path to forgiveness,' I say.

'That's so stupid. How are the police gonna help him?' G says.

I say, 'The philosopher Julia Kristeva says it makes sense that Dostoyevsky made art to channel the preoccupation with forgiveness. We make art because we are seeking transformation and freedom. These are the same reasons we forgive.'

Tommy puts his art folder down by the side of his chair and folds his arms.

'Forgiveness entails telling an old story in a new way that no longer burdens you. Art, like forgiveness, is achieved through the imagination. This is why Kristeva says that art can be a form of mercy.'

'If that was true, then Caravaggio wouldn't have had to send the picture to Rome,' Tommy says. 'He could have just painted it and then forgiven himself.'

'But Caravaggio could just forgive himself though,' G says.

'There's not a canvas in the world big enough for him to be able to do that,' Tommy says.

'But people do it all the time. I've heard loads of people say they've forgiven themselves,' G says.

'It can't be your hand that signs off on your own forgiveness,' Tommy says.

G yawns and stretches again.

'All you can do is accept what you've done and try to find a way to forget it,' Tommy says.

'How long till this lesson is over? I need to sleep,' G says.

★

Ten minutes later, G is making a case for Caravaggio again.

'Come on, it could just as easily have been Tomassoni who killed Caravaggio in that duel,' G says.

'But it wasn't,' Tommy says.

'Caravaggio painted himself with his own head cut off. Look how bad he's punishing himself. He's earned the right to forgive himself,' G says.

'He made a hole in the world where life used to be. That should put a hole in him forever. He can forgive himself for being so destructive to himself, but that's all. Once you've done something like kill another person, then your life is out of your hands.'

'What even is the definition of forgiveness, anyway?'

'Forgiveness is when your view of someone isn't purely shaped by the bad they've done,' Tommy says.

'So that means we can forgive ourselves. We can see ourselves as more than just criminals. Don't you see yourself as more than just a criminal?'

'I'm too old for that,' Tommy says.

I lean forward and rest my elbows on the table.

I ask Tommy, 'Is Caravaggio too old to look at his life differently?'

'Caravaggio has put himself in the painting as a boy, but that's a lie. He isn't a boy any more. He's grown up and killed someone.'

I ask G, 'Is Caravaggio trapped by what he's done? Or could art offer him a way out?'

'If parole look at your record and see you've been going to art or writing and stuff then they're more likely to let you out,' G says.

Tommy says, 'Drawing a picture or writing a book don't mean you can forgive yourself, but it can make you more forgivable.'

G tuts. 'That's what I said.'

Tommy continues, 'Forgiveness happens in real life. There's a wall between real life and art. Making art might take you right up to that wall, but it won't take you over it. Kristeva is almost right – making art is the closest you can come to redemption without actually being redeemed.'

'Why do you draw then?' says G. 'Why do you sit in your cell and draw when you could just watch TV or play cards or smoke weed?'

'To be someone else.'

A few weeks later, I'm in my nan's living room, sat next to Frank on the sofa. Repeats of old nineties sitcoms play on the TV. Nan puts a plate with four Cherry Bakewells on the coffee table in front of me. I hold a mug of water on my lap. Frank tells the story of when he was a teenager and the police tried to prise his fists open so they could get his fingerprints on a cash box. When he laughed so hard in court, the judge thought he was crying and gave him a concurrent sentence. When he used to go for 'a night out' in his cell. When police wearing helmets and carrying shields surrounded his van and he, Vinnie and Carl stepped out of the car and an officer said, 'Sarge, they're pensioners.'

'Eat them cakes up, Andy. Or I've got some chocolate biscuits if you want,' Nan says.

'I'm not hungry, Nan,' I say.

'You'll waste away,' she says.

I sip from a glass of water.

Frank reaches into the pocket of his hoodie and takes out a pouch of tobacco and some cigarette papers. A nature programme comes on the TV. A white owl glides through a clear sky.

'When I was fourteen and egging along the coast, I came back with an owl's egg. It was perfectly round and white, like a gobstopper,' Frank says.

'What happened to your egg collection?' I ask.

'I kept them in a glass box I had made especially. When I got nicked, I gave it to a mate to look after for a couple of years. But his kids found them in his cupboard. They thought they were toys.'

He sprinkles some tobacco inside a cigarette paper. On the telly, an owl bobs its head from side to side.

'I regret egging,' Frank says.

'Really?' I say.

'I was killing unborn birds, wasn't I? I wasn't strangling them, but I was stopping them from having a life.'

I grin, waiting for him to make a joke about dead birds.

He carries on. 'I learnt the coastline by egging. It took me on an adventure. All them old East End burglars and bank robbers you see on the wing in prison, all of us started out egging.'

My grin fades.

'I missed those beautiful places when I was locked up. It was hard not being able to go there.'

Frank holds his unrolled cigarette paper on his lap.

'But you get used to it. You can get used to anything, that's what I've learnt. It doesn't matter what happens to you; you can take anything.'

I open my mouth, about to say, 'Those beautiful places are still there. Let's go there, Unc.' But I stop myself.

'It would have been better to just find a nest with no bird in it and take a picture of the eggs with a camera. I should have just left it at that,' he says.

I look at him and he gives me a pained smile. This is our clear day.

He licks the edge of the cigarette paper and rolls it closed.

Home

> The bigness of the world is redemption.
> REBECCA SOLNIT

I arrive at the prison at 7.20 a.m. and linger outside the entrance. I look across the sky for signs of daybreak, but there's only the orange haze made from street lights against the dark sky. Once, I stood in the doorway of a man's cell that had no photos of family or kids or lingerie girls on the walls, only a cut-out from a newspaper of an image taken from the Hubble Space Telescope. The paper was frayed at the edges from where he'd torn it out because he was not allowed to use scissors. The image was teeming with tiny bright swirls and stars, yellow and blue and white. It was stuck a few inches above his pillow. The photo captured only a tiny patch of the amount of sky he could see from his cell window, yet it contained over a hundred thousand galaxies.

A security officer, around my age, comes out of the front gate and smokes a cigarette a few feet away from me. He blows out his smoke and says, 'You waiting for someone to escort you in?'

'I've got keys. By the time I finish at five it'll be dark again.'

He joins me in looking at the sky. 'I suppose.'

'Don't you miss the daylight, working all day in prison in the winter?'

He takes a drag on his cigarette and says in a nasal voice,

'I'm going to Morocco next month.' He blows out his smoke. 'Doing a desert safari.'

'Staff training?'

He laughs. 'Last year I went to Egypt and saw all the coral. It was a million miles from this place. I'm earning almost double what I was on in retail. This year I'm going to see what the desert looks like.'

'What can you see on a desert safari?'

'Cactuses. Bats. They make you do the whole thing on a camel. You don't have the sea like with the beach but cos the sand is so white you tan quicker. The sun bounces up at you.'

He takes another drag of his cigarette. I say goodbye and go into the prison.

Thirty minutes later, I'm moving through the heart of the prison. Through the bars of the door, I see a dozen men lining up. They've been unlocked early so they can receive their morning methadone, Subutex, antidepressants or other medications.

Larry is in the line, an ex-student of mine. He's a skinny man with uneven facial hair. He spent thirteen years serving in the army before becoming homeless and then ending up in prison. Around one in ten men inside are armed forces veterans, swapping one regime for another. Newbrooke, an officer with a thick neck and a clean white shirt, monitors the queue. He wears a yellow and red crest on his shoulder, known as a tri-service badge, to indicate he's ex-military.

I go through the door and lock it behind me. I shake Larry's hand and we bump shoulders.

'I haven't seen you in a while,' I say.

'I was away on business,' he says.

'Is that so?'

'New York, Milan, Paris, C-wing,' Larry says.

Newbrooke calls Larry to collect his meds. Larry says goodbye, goes to the counter and is handed a small white paper cup with pills in it. He puts them in his mouth and swallows. Newbrooke steps towards him. Larry opens his mouth.

Newbrooke looks inside. 'Lift your tongue.'

Larry's arms hang limp.

'Clear,' Newbrooke announces.

The two men exchange banter for a few seconds. Larry steps to the side where a queue forms for men to be taken back to their cells.

I walk further down the landing and stop to knock on Stuart's cell door. I take out from my folder his certificate for completing the philosophy course. Stuart comes to the viewfinder. It's wide enough for me to see the central third of his face. He looks grey with sleepiness. I slide the certificate under his door.

'More wallpaper,' Stuart says.

He goes to his sink, picks up a tube of toothpaste and dabs the top onto the four corners of the back of the certificate. Blu-Tack is prohibited in prisons for fear men might use it to take an impression of a key or block the keyhole of the door.

He turns and sticks the certificate on his wall. I crane my neck to see the sides of his cell through the inspection hatch. He has almost entirely covered his wall with certificates from education courses and programmes for drugs counselling and anger management. He has found a way to live in what *is* and what *can be* at the same time.

A few minutes later, in my classroom, I set up the chairs in a circle. I write 'Home' on the board and wait, expecting the officer to call free flow any minute now.

Fifteen minutes later, there has been no mention of free flow. I straighten my pens on the table and move my notebook so it squares with the right angle of the corner of my desk.

Twenty minutes later, the room is still empty. The corridor outside is quiet too. Forty-five minutes after the lesson was supposed to start, a message comes over the radio that there's a lockdown, meaning all classes and non-essential activity are cancelled for the day. Men with kitchen jobs will be unlocked, but education, association in the yard and non-emergency healthcare appointments won't happen. The men will spend around twenty-three and a half hours of the day in their cells today. They will have half an hour to collect their food, make a phone call and shower, although the queues will likely be too long for many to do all three.

Unplanned lockdowns like this can happen when there's a security issue, like a big fight on the landing. An attempted escape at another prison can cause a butterfly effect whereby governors become hypervigilant and call a lockdown. The reason there is no movement today is because there aren't enough staff in to run the prison securely. The prison is overcrowded. Recruitment and retention of guards is an ongoing issue in the service. Burnout is high and people phone in sick a lot. Last year, I was working in a high-security prison where the staff numbers fell so much that classes were cancelled three or four days a week for the whole of December. On the days classes did run, students were sleepy and snappy. Many of them were desperate for me to give them extra reading so they could take it back to their cells, worried they wouldn't get let out again the next day.

The number of officers here is borderline for running a full regime. This morning there has been a road incident two miles away that has caused a build-up of traffic. Staff cannot get here in time for free flow and so a lockdown has been called.

Lockdowns make me feel dreary and defeated. Where my classroom could be the location for 'two-hour holiday', today the chairs will remain empty.

I pack my folder into my bag. I wipe the word 'Home' off the board and leave.

A few days later, I'm sitting in the armchair in my brother's living room. Dean is showing me his dance moves. My brother is out, but his partner Laura is here sitting on the arm of the sofa. She has large hoop earrings and a tea towel over her shoulder.

Laura hands me a children's introductory algebra book. I flick through the pages. The exercises are aimed at children of about nine or ten.

'It was only 20p in a charity shop,' says Laura.

'Why algebra?' I say to Laura.

'Do you think he's too small for it?'

'Six is a bit young.'

'But I'm seven in eleven weeks and four days,' Dean says. He switches on a tablet, walks up to me and puts it in my lap, so it is facing him. He's using me as a TV stand.

'Tell your uncle what eight times eight is,' Laura says.

Dean shrugs. 'Sixty-four.'

'He'll be doing algebra in no time,' Laura says.

Dean taps the tablet to play a video. I look down at the screen and see an avatar with a pumpkin head and silver boots. It swings its hips dancing. Dean steps back and swings his hips too.

'How's work?' she says.

'My housemate thinks I have a weed addiction. I come home some days with the smell in my hair,' I say.

'That happened when we had lots of people on day release. They were a nightmare for smuggling drugs back in.'

'They've installed body scanners in security now.'

'Fancy. Only thing that changed when I was there was the colour of the paint on the walls.'

Laura used to be a security officer in prisons, including one of the prisons I work at. She often did nights and weekends for the extra money, which made it hard for her to maintain relationships with people who didn't work in prison. Twelve years into her career, she was working in a prison for teenagers and tried to break up a fight between four boys in the chapel. She got caught in the middle of it and got pushed to the ground. The boys kicked her in the head, face, ribs, kidneys and stomped on her hands. Seven or eight other boys ran over to join in.

A few days later, she was in her bed, taking codeine for the pain. She looked through her contacts on her phone for someone to call, but almost everyone was another officer. She put her phone away and took another codeine to get to sleep.

The prison didn't want staff coming in if they had bruises on their face. It was said to disturb the boys or make some of them excitable. Laura waited for the purple marks around her eyes to fade and then returned to the landing. But she felt on edge. She hadn't been able to see the faces of all the people who attacked her, so now when she was talking with a boy, she didn't know if he had been one of the ones to stomp on her. With each shift, she became more and more anxious, until a week later she woke up one morning and stayed under the duvet. She'd lost her nerve.

She stopped going to work. Each day she took more codeine to manage the unease.

A few years later, she joined a recovery group, which is where she met my brother.

Dean spins three hundred and sixty degrees.

'Would you ever go back?' I ask Laura.

'If I had a job that meant I was just in a room and didn't have to see any of the prisoners. Or see the other officers. And I didn't have to have an emergency radio going off in my ear every two minutes or go running onto the wings when someone sounds the alarm. I could just be in a room, just with papers and the names, typing them on the computer to say they went to a workshop or got their medication. If I didn't have to see it all but could just tick "yes so-and-so had a visit", "so-and-so got released", then I'd do it. I'd just draw the blinds and stay in my chair.'

Dean punches both fists above his head.

Laura continues, 'The boys knew when you were just about to clock off. If you finished at 2 a.m. they'd press their alarm five minutes before and I'd have to go there and they'd tell you they were sick or suicidal, or they would have started a fight with their cellmate, just so I wouldn't leave.'

'I don't know how you survived it.'

'Most of them would call me mum by mistake.'

Both Jason and Laura spent over a decade of each of their lives in prison, albeit on different sides of the door. Their relationship is predicated on a story of shared recovery from that period and they almost never talk about prison together. They both look back on their respective pasts with a sense of lost time and wasted potential. When Dean was eighteen months old, Jason and Laura bought him a child's laptop, despite the fact it was meant for kids aged three and over. The corner of their living room floor is stacked with educational toys and books that are a few years ahead of Dean's age.

A decade ago, my brother re-entered my life while I was still grieving his loss. He became present, but I only knew how to love him in his absence. The last time I saw Jason was a few months ago, when we had milkshakes in McDonald's together and he was relieved to hear that I'd got high. My sobriety always reminded him of how much his addiction had affected me. 'Looking at you made me feel guilty,' he said. I'd got high in Lisbon because I wanted to unburden myself, but it turns out it was unburdening for him too.

'Would you take it again?' Jason asked me.

'I'm still in the discovery of having taken it. Everything I look at has a freshness about it,' I said.

'I wish you'd done it with me. I don't mean now, but when you was younger. If I'd been there more.'

'Your doses would've killed me,' I said.

'I'd have looked after you, if everything had been different.'

'I'm happy you've got your boys and Laura and that you've made a home, Jason.'

'Cheers, Bruv. I'm not doing too bad,' he said.

I stirred the milkshake with the straw. I remembered Andros saying, 'Eat a McDonald's for me,' and how I had never known what to say back.

'But I sometimes feel guilty too,' I said.

Jason's facial expression hardened.

'I'm sorry,' I said.

Jason put his hand up as if to stop me. 'Thank you. Thank you for caring. But I don't want you to feel that way. You're not guilty of anything.'

I felt tears forming in my eyes. I sipped from the straw and kept the chocolate milk on my tongue for a moment to taste it.

I swallowed. 'Thank you, Bruv,' I said.

For most of my life I've felt that my being free and well meant I owed a debt to my brother. Over these last months I've been trying to picture my life without that debt. How could I live? Who could I be? I don't know the answers to these questions yet, but I sometimes find hints during moments of everyday pleasure. Recently, I've been more easily delighted by things like birdsong, the dappled light in the shadow of a tree and the smell of a fruit as I peel it in the afternoon. In those seconds, the world feels real. I wonder if the path I need to take is one marked by simple moments of enjoyment.

Jason and I may never be as close as I wished we could be when I was a teenager. But, today, he wants me to be free and I'm more able to see him beyond the boy in prison he once was. By both of us knowing happiness in our lives, we could be each other's forgiveness.

In my brother's flat, I'm sat in the armchair and Dean presses play on another video. The music starts and he jumps and twists three hundred and sixty degrees. Jason returns home and steps into the living room. He stands behind Dean, making sure he doesn't fall over.

Laura shouts from the kitchen. 'I showed Andy that algebra book. He reckons it's too advanced for him.'

'That will change in no time,' Jason says to me. 'Every day I watch him learn and grow. It's mad, Andy.'

The music crescendoes. Dean squats, touches his fingers to the floor and jumps up in the air.

A minute later, Jason takes off his hoodie and his T-shirt underneath rucks halfway up his belly. I see a scar tracing the curve of his hip bone.

The music fades out. Dean turns to his dad and puts his arms out for a hug. Jason pulls his T-shirt down and embraces his son. I feel a bubble of joy rising in my chest. I pick up my phone and take a picture of them together.

A few days later, I see Jerome on the landing, the man who was in my classes on Luck and Laughter. Since I last saw him he would have been released and so perhaps he has been recalled or reconvicted again. I wave to him across the landing. He gives me a big smile and waves back.

I walk down the twos and feel something fall on my head, something wet. I look up, expecting to see a young man on the threes holding a bottle of water and laughing at me. But I see no one, just drops of water falling through the metal anti-suicide nets that divide the landings. I walk on a few steps and come to a wide shallow puddle. The metal stairwell in front of me is soaking. Drips fall down and the water ripples.

Officer Newbrooke comes out of a door dragging a large empty bin across the landing and places it under the stairwell. He tells me a man on the fours has flooded his cell as a protest. A drop falls and makes a smacking sound, hitting the bottom of the plastic bin. I tread through the puddle and up the stairs.

I go to my classroom, set up the chairs in a circle and feel a buzz of anticipation as I wait for the men to arrive. An officer in the corridor shouts, 'Free flow,' and the men trickle in to my room. Harry arrives. He's in his mid to late twenties but has rosy cheeks and thin hairs on his top lip, like a schoolboy. He hardly ever says anything. As far as I'm aware the only person who comes to visit him is a youth worker who has known Harry since he was fourteen.

During the last class, the Albanian, Vietnamese and Colombian men were gathered around the map on the wall at the back of the classroom. They were showing each other where they came from; one man found his exact city and marked it by pressing his fingernail into it. After they'd gone back to their chairs, Harry walked over to the map and tried to find where he was from. Harry is English. He circled the Indian Ocean with his finger. He knew England had water around it. He brushed his finger from Brazil to Indonesia.

I pointed at England for him.

'Oh yeah. I thought it was th–' He swallowed the last word.

Harry spends the best part of his days in a six-by-eight

cell. I wonder how big his world was before he came to prison, and how big it will be after he leaves.

The last few men come into the class, including a man called Anthony. After spending the last two years living on the streets, Anthony is doing his first jail now in his early thirties. He keeps all his clothes and possessions in a pile next to his bed, so that he could throw them into a bag in ten seconds should he get shipped to a different prison.

The men in the circle are speculating about whether there'll be another lockdown tomorrow. Someone sniggers. It's Easton. He's leaning on the edge of a table in the corner, at the back of the room. Easton wears tracksuit bottoms that he has cut off to the knees to make into shorts. He wears these even on cold days. He says full-length tracksuit bottoms make him feel claustrophobic. I've seen Easton's cell. He has no pictures up. There are only white blobs scattered across the wall from where the previous person had put pictures up with toothpaste.

I close the door and get the lesson underway.

I say, 'The word nostalgia comes from the Greek *nostos* meaning "homecoming", and *álgos* meaning "ache". To be nostalgic is to be homesick. In the seventeenth century, soldiers diagnosed with nostalgia were deemed as unfit for duty and could be discharged. The Swiss army blamed homesickness on soldiers singing a Swiss song about milking cows. Any man who sang the song could be punished by death.'

'Priti Patel,' someone mutters.

'A Russian general buried two men alive because they said they had nostalgia. Doctors tried different methods to cure it. Some thought it came from a pathological bone in the body, however they never found it. Others tried leeches, purging the stomach, and warm hypnotic emulsions. A French doctor recommended that nostalgia should be treated by "inciting pain and terror". In the American military, a doctor advised that nostalgics be bullied for being unmanly and weak. Sometimes the doctor would recommend that to cure a soldier's nostalgia you could just send a man home, but even that wasn't guaranteed to work, if the home they longed for had changed.'

Anthony says, 'The homesickness I feel in my cell isn't for drugs or the street or the things I was actually wasting my time on when I was outside. It's for my nephews, the friends who haven't given up on me. Homesickness gives you clarity, helps you remember what's important.'

'So is homesickness a sickness?' I ask.

'Clarity is a cure, for the confusion. It puts things back in the right order. A sickness is something from nature, homesickness was invented by institutions like the military. Prison was an institution invented to make people homesick so that they'll change.'

'What are you saying?' Easton says, projecting his voice from the back of the room. 'Are you saying the homesickness we feel in here is good then?'

Anthony says, 'When they invented prison they didn't anticipate how you get used to it. My first day in prison I remember seeing the toilet right next to my bed in my cell and I could smell my cellmate's shit as I was lying on my bed. And at night it was so loud I didn't sleep. I swore to myself I'm never doing crime again. But after a week or two I could sleep. I've got used to the smell of shit.'

'What does that say about homesickness?' I ask.

'You get used to the homesickness too,' Anthony says. 'When I think of home I don't really miss it; it's like I remember it in my head and not my body, like the memory is hollow.'

A few minutes later, Easton slides off the edge of the table and stands up.

'Say man is banged up for fifteen years,' he says. 'He does every day of it behind the door. In jail he knows the barber, knows everyone on his landing, everyone in the gym.'

He stands with his feet wide apart. He points at me with his first two fingers, his hand the shape of a gun.

'Then man gets out,' he says. 'First night outside is harder than his first night inside. Knows nobody on his tower block. Nobody says hello. He can't get a job. The tempo inside was slow and now, outside, life is flying past him.'

Easton walks the width of the classroom floor.

He carries on. 'When he hears the sound of keys he feels less anxious. Man doesn't know what to do all day but looks at the time and knows it's half eleven so that'll be free flow, or it's after six so they'll be on bang-up.'

He turns and paces another width of the room.

'In bed man can't sleep because it's too quiet.'

He turns on his heel, his trainers squeaking on the floor. He keeps pacing.

'Someone bumps into him on the tube platform and doesn't say sorry and he thinks, "If you knew, mate, if you knew what I was in for" – nobody would diss him like that on the landing. In the end man misses jail, gets nostalgic for jail, wants to go back.'

He paces another width. I'm reminded of Nietzsche's

imperative to 'Sit as little as possible; do not believe any idea that was not born in the open air and of free movement.' I wonder how a man locked in here is able to tell which of his thoughts he should trust.

Easton continues, 'Nostalgia ain't an illness, but nostalgia for jail, that's illness.'

'If you are homesick for prison that means prison has become your home,' Anthony says.

Easton takes a couple more strides, points at Anthony with his two fingers. 'Being homesick for prison is missing something sick.'

'So if homesickne—'

'Man that misses jail isn't *home*sick, he's sick-sick.' He stops in the corner of the room and turns to me. 'Prison's not *my* home, *I* don't live here.' He jabs two fingers in the middle of his own chest. 'This isn't me. Me is who I am on the outside, me is who I'll be when I leave.'

A few minutes later, Pap is talking, a man in his mid-twenties from Malaysia whose front four teeth are gold. 'This would never happen in my country,' he says. 'Where I come from, if you do something wrong they cane you until you bleed. Nobody gets homesick for jail. They beat you because they care. Here, they don't give a fuck about you. They don't even care enough to punish you properly. Then people actually miss prison. How fucked up is that?'

'You sound like the doctor who said use pain on the soldiers,' Anthony says.

'It worked, didn't it? If you want people to not want to go inside then make prison harder.'

'Sounds like you're homesick,' Anthony laughs. 'You nostalgic for the beatings?'

'I'm telling you, this prison is too soft,' Pap says.

I tell the men to talk amongst themselves. Groups mutter to each other. Easton sits down in the circle next to a young man who lives on the twos with him. They're laughing together conspiratorially. During association two weeks ago, a few minutes before the guards were about to call bang-up, Easton and a dozen other young men from the twos went upstairs to the fours. They lingered at the far end of the landing, the furthest possible distance they could be from their own cells. It bought them another fifteen minutes, as that was how long it took the guards to usher the crowd back down to the twos. Easton and the boys did the same for the next few days, so last week the officers announced bang-up fifteen minutes early to get Easton locked up at normal time. The next day Easton and his mates went up to the fours twenty minutes earlier to stay ahead of the game. But the more Easton tried to get more time out of his cell, the more the regime took time away. Yesterday the officers called bang-up thirty minutes earlier than scheduled, halfway through association.

Harry is slumped in his chair, his hands in his pockets, staring into space. I say, 'What do you think, Harry?'

He screws up his mouth.

'Is homesickness a sickness?' I say.

'I don't know really.'

'What about Pap's idea? Should prison be harder?'

'I don't know. I don't know really.'

There are many people like Harry in prison, who never

know what to say or what they think, who are told when to eat, when they are allowed to go into the association yard and when they have to come back into the building. Men whose doors only lock from the outside and who speak in wispy voices that trail off.

An hour later, an officer bangs on the door to call time. Anthony slaps his belly, ready for dinner. The men leave. A man I've never seen before comes up to my room and says, 'Teacher, you help me.' He unfolds a piece of paper to show me; it's grubby and torn in the creases. 'Bail, please!' He points at the box on the form that lists his own address. It is blank but for the first two letters of his postcode.

'What's your name?' I say.

In broken English he tells me that he's trying to get bail but he cannot remember his own address. He has his landlord's number and has tried calling him to find out the address but the calls always go onto the answer machine. He has run out of the credit he has on his prison phonecard trying to call his landlord. 'Can you call him?' he says.

I look at his ID and see the name Florin. I say, 'Florin, what is your address?'

He hits his head with the heel of his hand and says he doesn't remember, that he was drinking a lot and only lived there for a few months. He recalls the door number was either 29 or 31 or 39. I ask if he knows his housemates so he can contact them and he says, 'One Poland, one Romania,' but he doesn't remember their names.

'So you want to get bail so you can go home?' I ask.

'Yes, please help,' Florin says.

'But to go home you need to know your home address

and you don't know your home address so you can't go home?'

'Yes.'

I tell him I cannot make calls on his behalf, but I write a note explaining his situation so he can pass it on to an officer who will help. He heads back towards his cell.

Thirty minutes later, I leave my class and walk down the corridor and come to the stairs of the landing. Water still drips down from the cell that was flooded this morning. There is water on the stairs. The normal rumbling sound of scores of people coming down the steps isn't there. Instead the men tread carefully, making small splashes.

I go down the staircase, check the bin and see it has gathered a few inches of water. A drip falls down my front and leaves a dark wet mark on my green shirt. I look up and see Easton and a group of young men on the fours, ambling past the yellow 'Beware of Slipping' signs.

Fine drops of water land on my forehead and nose. An officer walks towards Easton's group. The boys turn and head towards the other end of the fours.

Three more officers approach the group. Easton hangs his head and he and the boys amble towards the staircase.

A spot of water lands on my cheek.

A few weeks later, I'm in a bookshop and pick up a children's version of the story of Daedalus and his son Icarus. It tells of how the two are held captive on Crete by King Minos. There's a full-page illustration of them fashioning wings from chickens' feathers and golden-coloured wax so they can try and fly away from the island back to Athens where they come from. I buy the book and board a train to my brother's place.

The train pulls away. I look out of the window as we cross the Thames. London is bathed in the light of the pale winter sun. I think of Tommy, the draughtsman from my Caravaggio class, who drew teabags in his cell. If he were here he might notice the contrast between the white stone of St Paul's Cathedral next to the grey blue of the water; his attention might fall on the horizontal line of Blackfriars Bridge and the small boat motoring under it, leaving diagonal ripples in its trail. The city is more beautiful for looking at it on Tommy's behalf, savouring the landscape because he can't.

After the feeling of unreality I had on the train last year, I worried that my preoccupation with life inside prison was costing me the world outside. I had started to think that it might be time for me to finally look away. But meeting people in jail like Tommy, Andros and Yannis has enhanced my experience of the world. I can step out of the prison gate and appreciate things like beauty, food and friendship and not think of it as obnoxious towards those who live in deprivation, but rather as a way of staying connected to their humanity.

I don't want to look away. But I don't want to 'bear witness' either. A few weeks ago, I had a man in my class called Nick, who was doing a long sentence inside a single cell. He told me that sometimes he'd wake up in the middle of the night and feel a profound emotional and mental numbness that made him think he was not actually real. I've heard many people in prison express a similar anguish; they fear they are disappearing, not only from society, but from themselves. Once, at the end of a class, an officer knocked on my door to take the men back to their cells. The men filed out, but Nick came up to me.

'Philosophy is all right,' he said. 'It reminds me that I have a mind.'

The officer at the door said, 'Let's go.'

Nick held my gaze.

'Make sure you come back next week,' I said.

He nodded at me and went with the officer.

Nick reminded me that as a teacher, I can do more than bear witness to the vanished. I can help people keep sight of themselves.

An hour later, I arrive at Jason's and *Judge Judy* is playing on the TV. Jason is on the sofa eating a leftover fish finger from Dean's lunch. I give Dean the book and Laura says, 'What do you say?'

'I'm going to be seven in seven weeks and four days,' Dean says.

'You say, "Thank you, Uncle Andy,"' Laura says.

'Thank you, Uncle Andy. It's fifty-three days until my birthday,' Dean says.

On the screen, Judge Judy looks over the top of her glasses at the defendant who is arguing with her.

'She's gonna go to town on him,' Jason says.

'It's too late to argue,' says Laura.

Judge Judy declares the defendant owes $850 and he should learn how to count before he comes into her court again. The audience claps. Jason and Laura look at each other and laugh.

A few minutes later, I'm sitting on the sofa. Jason's misshapen green jumper is scrunched up on the arm next to me. I fold it neatly and put it back. Today I find Jason's possessions strangely affecting. I brush my thumb over his TV remote control that's held together with Sellotape and I trace the edges of his tobacco tin with the pad of my finger, enjoying the tactile confirmation that he is here.

'Let me show you this!' Laura says to me. I sit on the sofa next to my brother and watch her unroll a large world map she tells me she found for a pound in a charity shop. She leans it slanted against a wall, the edges curling, and she says, 'Where's Mexico?'

Dean stabs his finger at the orange blob below the USA.

'Indonesia?' Laura says.

He skips to the side and points at Indonesia.

'Don't cry for me Argentina?'

'You're only doing the easy ones,' Dean says and points at Argentina.

'All right, Mr Know-it-all,' Jason says, and clears his throat of the fish finger he's just eaten. 'Where's Iceland then?'

'There,' he says, lazily pointing at Iceland.

'Mongolia?' Laura says.

Dean looks at the map from left to right.

'Got you, haven't I?' Laura says.

He steps closer to the map, peering at Africa.

'You don't know where Mongolia is,' Laura says, teasingly.

Dean holds his head with both hands.

Laura points at Mongolia.

'Ahhhhh!' He jumps up and down. 'I knew it was there!'

'No you didn't,' Laura says.

'Ask me again. I knew it was there, ask me again.'

Kindness

We wanted to confess our sins but there were no takers.
White clouds refused to accept them, and the wind
Was too busy visiting sea after sea.
We did not succeed in interesting the animals.
Dogs, disappointed, expected an order,
A cat, as always immoral, was falling asleep
A person seemingly very close
Did not care to hear of things long past.

CZESŁAW MIŁOSZ

I haven't been in a prison for a year, since the pandemic started. Some of the inner-city prisons I work in have been keeping people in their cells for twenty-three hours a day, except for those who get out to clean the landing or work in the kitchen. The death rate has been three times higher inside than outside. Wayne, the IPP student who was in my class about *Waiting for Godot*, was due to have his hearing nine months ago, but it has been put on hold. He doesn't know when it will happen. My former student Sofia is also trapped. Sofia went to prison a few weeks after arriving from Romania as a teenager, only able to speak a handful of words in English. In the ten years she's been inside, she's done a degree in English. At the end of 2019, she was told she would be released. It would happen in increments. For the first year she would be allowed out in the day to go to university and return to prison in the evening. In the elation of getting this news, she asked me, 'Do I have a London accent?' She had only ever spoken English in prison. She wasn't confident about how to place her own voice.

'A little bit,' I said.

'So I might fit in?' she said.

Sofia's release has been put on hold. She doesn't know when it will restart.

A few men have been writing to me from their cells, sharing their thoughts on freedom, time and hope. The letters are often difficult to read because they have so many wrong spellings. It's hard for people to get hold of a dictionary right now. I write letters back, which the officers slide under the men's doors. A friend of mine who is an officer told me, 'I don't know how much longer I can take it. Every day I go in, and the men are out of reach. You can't really be there for them when they are rotting behind a cell door. I know this sounds strange, but I can't handle the bang-up.'

A writer I know called Steve Newark has done a total of about fourteen years in prison. He was inside when Covid hit, but is out now. I spoke to him on the phone last night. He said a lot of men on the wing were saying it wasn't fair that they weren't getting visits and were being banged up for so long. 'I didn't have time for that. You have to deal with the situation you're in rather than the one you want to be in.' Hearing him say that, I felt humbled by his ability to focus in dire circumstances. He was released whilst restrictions were at their highest. 'I felt like I didn't know what to do,' he told me. 'Everyone on the out had learnt how to adjust to lockdown together. I wasn't sure if I was supposed to wear a mask in the street, when I was supposed to queue or not – it felt a bit like my first ever day in prison.' Since he's been out, several people have said to him, 'I know what it's like for you in prison now.' I felt irritated on Steve's behalf that people would say something so blithe to him. I asked him if it annoyed him when people said that. 'I just smile and move on,' he said. 'People only know what they know.'

Two months into lockdown, the executioner closed in on me. I woke up at 2 a.m., my body crushed with panic. Castigating thoughts played in my head on a loop. This happened every night for almost a week, until every corner of my mind was taken up by shame. Throughout the day there was no space to have a thought that was not mortifying. I felt short of breath, like I was going to faint.

The following week, I started running in a large park, but after a few days I noticed how all my runs were around the same hundred-square-metre patch of grass. When I looked at my fitness app, my heat map was a small red circle. The image showed something constricted, monotonous and joyless, which is what the inside of my head looks like under the executioner. It was as though he was plotting my route for me. The next day I ran in random zigzags across the same park. But that frightened the dogs. They kept barking at me.

Now I just leave my front door and run in whichever direction I feel like. At first, punishing images flash into my mind. But I keep running. The wind hits my face and scatters my thoughts. By the time I remember what the image was, I've already turned onto a new street. I run until I cross a threshold where the thoughts stop. I feel the air coming into my mouth and filling my lungs; the red bricks of the houses look more vividly red; the world becomes bigger than my alleged guilt. At those moments I'm neither running to the executioner, nor running away from him. I am just running.

I've gone back to reading Kafka. As usual, I wasn't sure if that was a step towards or away from the executioner. But I recently found a moment where Kafka allows a character some kind of escape. He takes the story of Prometheus, how he was chained to a mountain and the gods sent eagles that ate at his liver as it kept growing back, but Kafka suggests an alternative ending. 'In the course of millennia . . . everyone grew tired of the procedure, which had lost its raison d'être. The gods grew tired, the eagles, too. Even the wound grew tired and closed.' At first it was too late for Prometheus, but then it no longer is. I wondered if Kafka was telling us that he had finally become tired of his own torture. Had he found liberation by becoming bored of his symptoms? If I keep reading his work, could I find liberation by becoming bored of Kafka?

Perhaps the quickest way to exhaust my interest in the executioner is to become interested in other things. A few nights ago, in the hours before I got into bed, I put a random radio station on. It was a pre-emptive measure against the executioner's droning repetition. They played tracks from Miles Davis, Ella Fitzgerald and Ahmad Jamal. I listened to the melodies, wanting to refamiliarize myself with surprise in the hope it would keep my thoughts from narrowing so gruesomely in the night. Although pre-empting my anxiety is sometimes the very thing that summons it, listening to new music made me excited about life. That's one way of not going to the executioner.

In the summer, I stayed with Adam in Lisbon for a week. During the second night, I lay awake and kept having the same condemning thought each minute. In the morning I had a headache, as if my brain was sore from treading the same synapses over and over again. The next day, Adam took me to a forest. We lay down and we took some magic mushrooms. Thirty minutes later, the trees took on the aura of kings and queens. I wanted to show them respect, but a leaf near my face kept making me laugh. Everything around me became interesting. It was as if I could feel my entire brain lighting up. I couldn't have gone to the executioner even if I'd wanted to; I was too interested in what it felt like to slowly rotate my ankle.

I'd always avoided psychedelic drugs for fear I'd lose control and do something violent, that when I came down I'd find blood on my hands and realize the executioner was right all along. But I didn't hurt anyone. I just had a really fun time. The day after taking mushrooms, I allowed myself to enjoy a provisional feeling of calm. Perhaps, I thought, I might be able to trust myself. Perhaps the decades I'd spent under the executioner had been a painful waste of time. I appointed that draconian figure in my head to make sure I never became like my dad, but in reality, the only thing the executioner has done is stop me from being myself. That night, I got into bed and told myself that if the executioner comes for me, I will tell him he has the wrong person.

For the last few weeks, I've been dating a translator called Iona. She told me that one day during the winter months of lockdown, she spontaneously gathered her books, clothes, sofa cushions, candleholders and other items into dozens of black bags and got rid of them. She felt relieved about having created more space but, a few days later, she felt hemmed in again. She decluttered vases, excess cutlery, rugs, pictures from the wall, chairs, storage boxes and pens. At night she sat on her sofa to relax but felt there were more things she could clear out.

I went to hers for the first time last week. We sat in her living room and she read me passages from some of her favourite novels, translating them into English as she spoke. We made love and fell asleep there on the sofa, with books and clothes scattered on the floor.

In the morning we woke up and she rested her head on my chest. I felt a twinge of dread. The executioner told me I deserve to have everything taken off me. I put my arm around Iona. It felt so daring.

We got up together and made tea in her kitchen. I opened the fridge and saw that she had several packets of cheese that were four months out of date. Next to them were three unopened cans of beans.

'You don't need to keep tinned food in the fridge,' I said.

She shrugged.

'I don't want you to eat this cheese,' I said.

'Food is for wimps, anyway.'

'One thing you should know about me is that I need to eat in the morning before I do anything.'

'Well, my day doesn't go well unless I'm wearing lipstick.'

In the economic turbulence of the pandemic, Iona's days are very long. She has been working at her desk late into the night, flamenco red lipstick on her mouth and the blue light of her laptop shining onto her face. She occasionally stops to make cereal and brings it back to her desk to keep working while she eats.

I'm at home. It's Sunday, around midday. My mouth is dry. I fill a glass with water under the kitchen tap and drink it. I'm enjoying the pleasure of having my thirst quenched, but then an image appears in my head. I am locked in a chamber. There isn't enough space to move my arms. My mouth is dry and I have no water. I am passing out from dehydration. The executioner tells me I deserve it.

In the kitchen, I set the glass down on the counter. I take out my phone and make a video call to Johnny. He picks up and I see he is sat in his garden, beneath a eucalyptus tree. We talk for a few minutes. I still feel clouded by darkness, but somehow I trust it less. The image of the chamber is still somewhere in my mind, but I can't hold on to the thought.

'Are you OK? How are you coping with lockdown?' he says.

'I've been writing,' I say.

'Something funny?'

'It's about prison.'

He tuts. 'You.'

I smile. I sip my water.

Throughout lockdown, at moments when I have almost lost myself to shame, I've been able to pick up the phone to a friend who has reminded me who I really am. Meanwhile in prison, people have not been allowed visits. The social and sensory deprivation is eroding people's sense of personhood. This morning I listened to some recordings of people in prison on the *Inside Time* website. One man called David said, 'Sometimes you look forward to the door opening for your food, just so you can speak, even though you're only saying, "Thank you", you've got to make sure your voice still works, haven't you?'

An hour later, I'm cycling to Iona's place and listening on my earphones to more recordings of David on the *Inside Time* website. 'You can't move,' he says. 'My kidneys and my body are hurting because you either have to lie down or sit in the chair for twenty-three hours a day and there's nothing you can do about it.'

I'm suddenly aware of the sensations of movement, speed and balance as I pedal.

I lock my bike up outside Iona's building, take out my earphones and cross the road to a grocers. I pick up an avocado, some tomatoes and a loaf of bread. In the aisle, I see a man with a bald head and dark eyes. His mask covers the bottom half of his face, but he looks like someone who used to be in my class. I meet his eye and smile before I realize he cannot see I'm smiling because of my mask. He turns to the side and seeing his profile I realize he's not the person I thought he might be. Many times over the last year, I've thought strangers were ex-students. I feel so powerless about not being able to see the men in jail that I keep thinking I can see them outside.

I join the queue to pay. The man behind the till stands beneath a harsh fluorescent strip light. He pulls his mask a couple of inches away from his face and wipes the sweat away from his top lip. He scans a customer's items and puts them in a blue carrier bag. The customer is scrolling on their phone. They have earphones in.

'13.42,' the shopkeeper says.

The customer takes out one earphone.

'13.42,' the shopkeeper says.

The customer taps their card on the machine and leaves. I come to the counter. The checkout worker scans and bags my items. I can see in his face how hard his job is right now. He works twelve-hour days, at risk of infection, packing the fruits and vegetables of Londoners who don't look at him.

'Thank you,' I say.

He looks me in the eye. 'Thanks,' he says.

I hand some cash through the hole at the bottom of the Perspex. He hands me my change. I step out of the shop and cross the street halfway and stand on the island in the middle of the road, waiting for the traffic to pass. Behind me, a car speeds over a pothole. It sounds like it's driving over a body. The executioner tells me that I don't really have any feeling towards the checkout worker. My care is fraudulent.

I step into the road. A driver coming towards me hits his horn and I step back onto the kerb.

He shouts at me through his window as he passes.

I stand on the island. Cars speed past both sides of me.

When the executioner alleges that I have burnt down the house or might hurt someone with a knife, I know how to not run to him. But then there are these moments where he tells me that I'm not capable of kindness. Of all of my dark thoughts, this is the one that makes me feel most alone. It's when the guilt feels most claustrophobic. I don't know how to escape it.

A few months before the pandemic started, I was locking up my bike in the prison car park. A prison van drove past me. The man inside was thumping the walls and shouting. Feeling ominous, I took out my phone and typed a message to Johnny. 'Are you free?'

I held my thumb above the send button. I couldn't shift the thought that I had to get through the dread by myself. I deleted the text and put my phone away.

Twenty minutes later, I was in my classroom, filling out

the form to update my security clearance. One question was, 'Have you ever had any criminal convictions? Please tick Yes or No.' Next to the 'Yes' box, I wrote that several years ago I got fined £20 for running through a red light on my bike.

Free flow started. Martin, a greying man with greasy hair and an unkempt beard, was the first to arrive to class. I could smell his body odour from two metres away. It was his first time in prison and he'd be doing a year and a half. Martin's grown-up son had come to visit him for the first time two days before, but Martin just stayed in his cell, too ashamed to let his son see him. He hadn't shaved since he arrived in prison about three months ago. He was always the first person to arrive to class, as if his punctuality was another part of his penance.

It's uncommon to see someone inside display as much guilt as Martin. A lot of people here see themselves as victims more than as perpetrators, which isn't surprising when you hear the stories of their childhoods. Those who do feel bad are so busy trying to survive the landing that they can only really engage with their remorse once they've been released. Martin looks so weighed down with shame. I worry how he will make it through his sentence.

A minute later, Billy and Kit walked in, arguing about who the sexiest woman on *Love Island* was last night. Billy had a receding hairline and thick chest hair poking out the top of his T-shirt, making him look ten years older than his actual age of twenty-three. Kit had salt-and-pepper hair and wore a red tracksuit top with the collar turned up. Billy thought the voluptuous Anna was the most beautiful. Kit thought it was the petite Jourdan.

Kit turned to Martin and said, 'Tell him I'm right. It's Jourdan.'

Martin didn't react.

'Have you seen that girl, Martin!' Kit says.

A stern expression was fixed on Martin's face.

Kit and Billy sat down on either side of Martin. Billy's nose wrinkled and he shuffled his chair back a few inches. Kit sat in the chair to Martin's right, seemingly unbothered by the smell.

A few minutes later, the class was underway. I drew a demon on the board.

I said, 'The philosopher Pierre-Simon Laplace said that if there was a demon who knew the precise location and momentum of every atom in the universe right now, then, using the laws of nature, it would be able to calculate where every atom would be tomorrow and for all the days after that.'

'That's deep,' Kit said.

'Humans are made of atoms. We're subject to the laws of nature. In theory, the demon would be able to look at a child and know precisely what they would be doing in thirty years' time as an adult,' I said.

'What about free will?' Kit said.

'If Laplace is right, then maybe we don't have free will.'

'Then no one should be in prison, if it's all just nature.'

'Yes. Our so-called choices are determined by earlier events, like our background and biology. Nobody would be truly guilty for what they do.'

'For your first offence, the judge takes into account your traumatic childhood when he's deciding how long to give you. But your second offence, they don't give a fuck about your past.'

'Should they?' I asked.

'For your second offence, the fact you've been to prison before should count as mitigating circumstances. Isn't this place traumatic too?'

'Do you think our lives are determined?'

'I think sometimes God can step in and change things.'

'Like what?'

'My lifestyle outside was chaos. My mum says if I hadn't been arrested, I'd be in the ground by now. She says me going to prison was divine intervention. It saved my life.'

Billy knew I also worked at a high-security prison not far from the prison he was in. He knew that because his dad was in custody there.

'What do you make of that place? Is it any good in there?' he asked me.

'I work there. I'm not really *in* there,' I said.

'My dad says it's organized. Unlock is unlock. Bang-up is bang-up. The regime here's chaos. They say they're gonna unlock you and then they keep you banged up all day. I'd much rather be over there.'

Because they were both in prison, it was difficult for Billy and his dad to talk on the phone. The phones on prison landings only call out. They cannot receive calls, so one prison payphone cannot call another prison payphone. When Billy and his dad wanted to talk, they had to go to the offices of their respective prisons and speak using the office line, whilst at both ends, guards stood monitoring the conversation.

I pointed to the demon on the board and asked Billy, 'Do you think that nobody is really guilty?'

'Everyone will take the piss if you say that,' Billy said.

'Don't you think our background shapes what we become?' I said.

'It'd be chaos if you didn't have prison. There has to be consequences.'

Martin's face was dark with rumination.

'What do you think, Martin? Are we responsible for where we end up?' I asked.

'I don't know who else could be responsible,' Martin said.

'Nietzsche said that moral responsibility was a harsh and unimaginative concept,' I said.

Martin sniggers.

'He thought we become preoccupied with guilt when our desire to punish ourselves is stronger than our desire for life. He said free will was the philosophy of the hangman.'

'And was Nietzsche a harm-causing individual?' he said.

'A what individual?' Kit said.

Billy sniggered and pulled the neckline of his T-shirt over his nose.

'Ain't everyone done something bad in their life? We ain't no different to people outside,' Kit said.

Martin folded his arms.

I said, 'What do you think, Martin? Is moral responsibility the philosophy of the hangman?'

'Nietzsche sounds like a very clever boy,' Martin said.

Conversations with Martin quickly reached a full stop. I'd ask him what he thought of various ideas and he'd say something that would shut the discussion down. Later on during that session, I said to the group, 'I think when you hold two thoughts in your head at the same time then something opens up.' I was directing my voice towards Martin, but his face remained stony. It was as though he thought it was too late for philosophy: no matter what he did or didn't think about this or that idea, he was in prison now.

When the class ended, I rubbed the drawing of the demon off the board. Martin came up to me on his way to the door and shook my hand.

'Thank you, Andy. It's so good of you to let me be here,' he said.

I laughed nervously. I didn't know what to say. It was as though his gratefulness to me was another act of self-reproach; I didn't want to be his accomplice.

'I really appreciate it,' he said.

I had to look away.

If Joseph K. lived in Laplace's universe, then no matter how many times he lived his life over, each time he walked down the street on that Sunday morning and paused to look at the world around him, he will always run to his trial. He will never escape his atomic fate.

Another philosopher, Lucretius, thought that it wasn't only atoms that were important, but also space. He recognized that there was space not just between objects but also within each object. There is space between two stones and within a single stone. Even within the most crushing boulder, there is space.

If Joseph K. lived in Lucretius's universe, then on that Sunday morning he could pause and feel the space between the street and the courthouse, between his guilt and the sight of someone savouring a cigarette, between his summons and his next step.

Lucretius thought that space was what allowed atoms to

move and that atoms could occasionally swerve from their trajectory. The material world wasn't always predictable. Sometimes it was spontaneous. For Lucretius, events could unfold in different ways. Joseph K. could turn away from the courthouse and walk in the other direction.

When I am in the most opaque panic, I am crushed with guilt and the executioner's voice takes up my entire head. But I think of Lucretius and remember that even the most singular thought has space within it. I let the executioner chatter on, as I slip away in between his words.

A few minutes after going to the grocers, I'm in Iona's kitchen, unpacking the food. The counter and stove are immaculately clean, as she hardly ever uses them. Iona is stood beside me, her glasses pushed up onto her head as she takes a break from work.

'That's so much food,' she says.

'It's not even a day's worth of food,' I say.

'What are you gonna do with it all?'

'I was going to put it in the fridge and let it go off,' I say.

She tuts. 'You're not funny. I'm going back to my desk.'

She stands behind me and watches as I cut the bread, lay two plates on the counter and put a slice of bread on each one. I cut open the avocado and squeeze out the flesh. Iona reaches around me and rests one of her hands on my chest. I feel the warmth of her belly against the small of my back.

'You're making two sandwiches,' she says.

'They are only for wimps though, I'm afraid,' I say.

I slice the tomatoes. Iona nuzzles her face in my neck. Her eyelashes tickle my skin as she blinks.

'I had another dream last night,' she says.

I rest the knife on the counter. Iona's mum died around this time a couple of years ago. She was also a translator. She and Iona used to speak to each other whilst going in and out of four or five different languages.

'I remembered it today when I was crossing the street,' she says. 'I never remember it until the daytime, when I'm walking down the street or I'm halfway across the road. That's when the grief hits me again.'

Her voice sounds like she is on the verge of crying.

She swallows and says, 'I'm talking so much. I need to work.'

I tear a small square of bread off the end of the loaf, turn around and hold it in front of her mouth.

'Go on. I promise I won't tell anyone,' I say.

She eats it. I stroke her face with the back of my fingers.

I turn around and continue making food. Iona rests her chin on my shoulder and watches. I add the tomatoes to the sandwich. I sprinkle on salt and pepper.

'Look at that. I almost feel like I'm in a restaurant again,' she says.

'I know, I'm feeling underdressed.'

'It would be fun to dress up.'

I turn around and face her. I hold my greasy hands close to my belly with my palms facing up, so I don't dirty Iona's clothes.

'I could wear a dress. You could wear a shirt,' she says.

She unbuttons the top two buttons of my shirt.

'Where would you take me?' I ask.

She touches the heel of my palm with her finger. 'Here. To the city.'

I raise an eyebrow.

She zigzags her finger across my palm. 'We'll walk through these narrow old streets where the buildings are made of stone. It's night, everyone is out and there's a stream of different faces. We can hear music coming from one of the basements. I take you by the wrist and lead you inside.'

I giggle bashfully.

She moves her finger to the very middle of my palm. I open my hand up a little more.

'We'll dance here all night,' she says.

I feel an obscure sense that I have done something wrong.

'When our legs are aching too much to dance any more then we'll go here,' she says, touching the skin where my palm meets my little finger, 'to the beach.'

Guilt squeezes me. I want this tenderness Iona is offering me, but I don't know how to acquit myself.

'We'll look at the ocean together,' she says.

I grimace. 'That's beautiful,' I say.

She squeezes my hand. 'Are you OK?'

'Yeah,' I say.

'Are you sure?'

'You have grease on your hands now,' I say.

I turn around, pick up the plates, and we go over to her sofa and sit with the food on our laps. Iona takes a bite of her sandwich and closes her eyes to enjoy the taste. The moment is tinged with a grim poignancy. The executioner tells me this meal is the last thing I will ever be able to give Iona.

Iona swallows her food and opens her eyes. She puts her hand on my knee. 'Thank you,' she says. 'This is so kind of you.'

I laugh nervously.

'What's funny?' she asks.

'I'm sorry,' I say, but I laugh again.

She takes her hand off my knee. 'Why are you laughing?'

The day after my class on Laplace's demon, I went into prison and told another teacher what I'd put on my security clearance forms. He burst out laughing.

'They don't need to know you ran a red light,' he said.

'I thought, what if they found out and I'd kept it a secret?'

'You're hilarious, Andy.'

'It's not that funny.'

I went to my classroom and got ready for my session. An officer in the corridor shouted, 'Free flow!' A few minutes later, Billy and Kit walked in. Kit was ranting about how he phoned his kids that morning and they'd told him they'd been on a day out to the Tower of London. 'Can you believe that's what they did instead of coming to visit me?' Kit said. 'They were telling me what the London Dungeon was like. I almost put the fucking phone down on them.'

The two men sat down. Billy told me he might miss our next class. 'I'm going for an assessment. I might get a twenty-five per cent discount on this sentence,' he said.

'A discount?' I said.

'You get twenty-five per cent off if they find you've got mental health. But you've gotta show up to the assessment.'

'Reckon you'll get it?' I asked.

'Fingers crossed,' he said.

Free flow ended. I stood in the doorway and looked down the corridor to see if I could see Martin, but I couldn't.

I asked Kit, 'Have you seen Martin?'

Kit shook his head.

'Do you know if he's OK?' I asked.
'Sometimes he just stays in his cell all day.'

I closed the door and took a seat opposite Billy and Kit.

'The philosopher Arthur Schopenhauer thought that life seemed like a form of punishment,' I said.

'Cheer up, Schopenhauer, it might never happen,' Kit said.

'Schopenhauer thought it was already happening,' I said. 'From the first day we are born, we suffer, even though we've done nothing wrong. He said it's tempting to think we come into the world carrying the guilt for our fathers' crimes.'

I tried not to look at Billy when I said 'fathers' crimes' but I ended up looking straight into his eyes when I said it.

I said, 'Schopenhauer thought that if you want to get by, you should think of this world as a prison. You won't get frustrated when people disappoint you because you'll understand they're also in the prison, trying to endure their punishment too.'

'When I get out of prison, I'm going for a drink, then a KFC, and then I'm eating a whole tub of chocolate ice cream and then I'm going to my girlfriend's,' Billy said.

'Does that mean Schopenhauer was wrong?' I asked.

'Schopenhauer needs to get laid,' Billy said.

I said, 'Schopenhauer said that if you think of the world as a prison, we'll treat each other with more tolerance, patience and kindness.'

Billy said, 'Prison makes you more tolerant, yes. More patient, yes. But kinder, no. You're more tolerant because you're sharing a cell with people you wouldn't be with normally, and you'll go fucking insane if you don't learn to let things go. You get more patient in jail, but that's not because you are kinder. It's because you've got loads of time on your hands.'

'Prison is where you learn what kindness means,' Kit said.

'Prison hasn't made me kind,' Billy said.

'People here are kind even though they got no reason to be,' Kit said.

'The last thing I'd want is for people on the landing to think of me as kind.'

'It don't matter what other people think of you.'

'If it gets around that I'm kind, people are gonna know they can come into my cell and take my stuff and I won't do anything back.'

A few minutes later, Kit said, 'If there's no kindness in prison, then how come there's not riots in here 24/7?'

'Because if you riot you get time added on to your sentence,' Billy said.

'What about the countless acts of camaraderie that happen automatically every day? Noticing that someone on the landing hasn't gone down for their dinner for a few nights and knocking their door to see if they're OK.'

'That's not really kind though, is it?' Billy said.

'Or what about letting someone use your phone credit because they need to call their kid. The Sunday cook-up where six of you put your fucking tasteless pieces of chicken together and one bloke puts in his herbs and another adds his spices and by the end of it you're all eating a kicking meal.'

'Yeah, but . . .'

'On the landing, I know people's names and whether they have sugar in their tea. I never knew that living in a tower block.'

Billy folded his arms. 'I just don't like the word "kind". It makes me sound like a weirdo.'

'I used to be the same. But now it's really important for me to notice the ways I'm kind, even if it's just in the smallest little thing,' Kit says.

'Why?' I asked.

'Cos I want to get out of this lifestyle,' Kit said. 'I'm never gonna change unless I can admit to myself that I can be a decent person.'

On Iona's couch, I apologize for laughing. For the next few minutes, I try to explain myself.

'An executioner?' she says.

'I mean, I don't literally mean Albert Pierrepoint is talking to me.'

'Well, whoever he is, I didn't enjoy meeting him.'

She looks down at her food. I pull my shirt closed over my chest.

She says, 'When I told you I thought this was beautiful, it felt cathartic. The words came out of my mouth and a tiny bit of my grief lifted.'

'I'm sorry. I don't want the executioner to claim that too.'

'Is he going to?' she asks. She searches my face.

Half an hour after my class with Kit and Billy, the officers were locking people up for the afternoon. I hurry down the landing to Martin's cell. His door was open. I looked inside and saw him. He'd shaved his beard off. His hair was fluffy from where he'd washed it.

'I'm looking for Martin. Do you know where he's gone?' I said.

He chuckled. 'I thought I best scrub up. I've arranged a visit with my son,' he said.

He smiled. There were the beginnings of tears in his eyes.

'I phoned him yesterday,' he said. 'I told him I understood if he couldn't forgive me for what I've put him through. He got angry with me. He said, "You're my dad. Forgiveness doesn't come into it."'

'He loves you,' I said.

'I know, I feel terrible about it. But I think it's gonna be OK,' he said.

An officer comes up to the door. 'I'm going to have to lock up, gentlemen,' he said.

I stepped back.

'See you in class,' I said.

The officer put the key in the door.

'He says he can come and see me once a fortnight. My time is going to go so much quicker if he's visiting me,' Martin said.

The officer pulled the door shut and locked it.

Martin and I waved goodbye to each other through the inspection hatch of his cell door.

Martin started coming out of his cell more after that. He ended up forming a close friendship with another middle-aged man on his wing. He applied for a job in the kitchen and got it. He worked in the day, passionately read books on his bed in the evening and the rest of the time he was looking into how he might work for a rehabilitation charity when he got out. He told me, 'I'm never bored in prison any more. Sometimes I don't have enough hours in the day.' From time to time, he still called himself 'greedy' or 'stupid' because of what he'd done. But despite his shame, he allowed space for other things in life too.

A few days after I told Iona about the executioner, I return from the shops to Iona's flat at midday and she is sat at her desk. She looks at the carrier bag of food in my hand and says, 'I want to eat in an hour.' I roll my eyes and go into her kitchen. I know that she wants my care, but she doesn't want to be disempowered by receiving it, so she asks me for it like she was giving an order. I unpack the vegetables from my bag. I wash them and make soup.

At lunchtime, I put her bowl on the dining table. Iona comes over.

'Beautiful,' she says. She touches my hip.

I feel a low hum of dread. But I put my hand over hers.

I used to think I couldn't receive Iona's tenderness until I'd found some way to clear my guilt. But I know the executioner is a stubborn occupant. It isn't workable to wait until he has gone for me to get on with my life. Instead, when I'm sharing a moment with Iona and I feel my insides tighten with guilt, I try to let myself feel her tenderness alongside the guilt. Even if I can't get out from under the executioner, I can allow space for Iona too.

We sit down and eat. I watch her finish her soup.

'I thought you said food is for wimps,' I say.

'I've realized I quite like being a wimp,' she says.

'I could cook something for us tonight.'

She looks into my eyes and says, 'You're sweet.'

I blink. I feel a lead weight of guilt in my stomach.

'Only if you can,' she says.
'I can,' I say.

I stay at Iona's for the week. She curses me for my habit of leaving my clothes on the floor and not picking them up until days afterwards. Epictetus said, 'If you hear that someone is speaking ill of you, instead of trying to defend yourself you should say: "He obviously does not know me very well, since there are so many other faults he could have mentioned."' This morning I wake up in Iona's bed to the executioner telling me I must have done something irredeemably bad. A few minutes later in the living room, Iona picks my shirt up off the floor and throws it at me. I laugh and say sorry. I am glad that Iona knows me better than the executioner does.

It was always too late for Joseph K. Kafka's past had determined K.'s future. I still get the thought that it's too late for me, but I also find myself excited about what it will be like to come out of lockdown with Iona. That excitement is my chance to turn away from the executioner and walk in the other direction. On the first warm spring day of the year, Iona and I are in the park, reclining on the grass under an ash tree, looking out on a lake. Friends, lovers and families with small children are sat around the edge of the water. A man steps from the grass onto a pontoon and takes a tarpaulin off several small rowing boats. All being well, he will rent them out again in the coming weeks.

Iona points up at the branches of the ash tree above our heads. I look up.

'Havina,' she says.

'What?' I say.

'It's Finnish. It describes the swaying of the branches.'

I gaze up and see the branches gently moving in the breeze.

'My mum taught me that word,' Iona says.

I look at Iona. 'Did you dream about her last night?' I ask.

Still gazing up, she smiles and shakes her head. 'I just thought of her now when I noticed how beautiful this tree is.'

I look back up.

'Habona,' I say.

'Hav-in-a,' she says.

'Havina.'

'That's it.'

Over the next hour, more people crowd around the lake. I hear the giggling of two children playing behind us. There is a crackle of excitement in the air. It feels like this might be the first day of the journey towards the city opening up. But the executioner tells me that I won't be joining everyone else on the walk to freedom. My breath becomes short. The guilt is smothering me.

A breeze comes. I look up and see the branches of the ash tree sway. The leaves flutter and brush against one another.

I let out a sigh.

'Havina,' I say.

'That's right,' Iona says.

A couple of months later, shops and restaurants are open. I'm told that we are still several months away from the regime returning to normal inside. I spoke to my uncle Frank yesterday. He told me that he took a spontaneous trip to

Sandwich. He took a state-of-the-art camera with him (a friend of his recently came into 300 of them). Today I'm going to see him. I wheel my bike out of Iona's building, onto the street. The ground is wet from where it has been raining. A double-decker bus with only two people on pulls over at a bus stop and one of them gets off. I get on my bike and ride down some backstreets.

A fine spray of water comes off the tip of the tyre. A tailwind pushes me forward. I freewheel and close my eyes to enjoy the sensation of moving without strain.

I open my eyes and turn onto a main road. A Deliveroo driver with a black mask over his mouth and nose cruises past me. I approach a traffic light that is turning red. I stop.

About twenty metres down the road, a police car is pulled over. On the pavement, a young man with acned cheeks stands with an officer on either side of him. He's in handcuffs. One officer opens the back door of the car and the boy ducks his head and goes inside. The officer shuts the door. The two police get in the front seats and one starts the engine. The orange indicator light flickers.

The car behind me beeps its horn. I look up. The traffic light has turned to green.

Classroom Materials and Sources

I've been so lucky to receive ideas and inspiration from my colleagues at The Philosophy Foundation over the last decade. Thank you to Peter Worley for his lesson plans on the Sirens, Epictetus, the Frog and the Scorpion, the Happy Prisoner, Diogenes and the Ship of Theseus. They are available in his books *The If Machine*, *The If Odyssey* and *40 Lessons to Get Children Thinking*, all from Bloomsbury Education. Thank you also to David Birch for his lesson on Pandora's Box, which is in his book *Thinking Beans*, from One Slice Books.

I developed the methodology I use for teaching in prisons with Mike Coxhead and Andrea Fassolas. Teaching alongside them, I learned so much from how perceptive, determined, generous and uncynical they were. They both helped to co-write materials on Hiroo Onoda, the cleansing of the temple, Simon Wiesenthal and moral luck.

List of Epigraphs
Marcel Proust, from *In Search of Lost Time*
Jean Genet, from *The Thief's Journal*
Simone Weil, from *Gravity and Grace*
Nâzım Hikmet, from 'Some Advice to Those Who Will Serve Time in Prison'
Franz Kafka, from *The Trial*

Fernando Pessoa, from *The Book of Disquiet*
Michael Ondaatje, from *The English Patient*
Primo Levi, from *If This Is a Man/The Truce*
John Berger, from *What Time Is It?*
Dostoyevsky, from *The Brothers Karamazov*
George Eliot, from *Daniel Deronda*
Telemachus, from Homer's *Odyssey*
Mary Boykin Chesnut, from *A Diary From Dixie*
Anaïs Nin, from *House of Incest*
Ocean Vuong, from *On Earth We're Briefly Gorgeous*
Milan Kundera, from *Testaments Betrayed*
Zadie Smith, from 'Fascinated to Presume: In Defense of Fiction'
Edward St Aubyn, from *Some Hope*
Alexander Pushkin, from a letter from Pushkin to Nashiokin (March 1834)
Samuel Beckett, from *Stories and Texts for Nothing*
Rebecca Solnit, from *The Faraway Nearby*
Czesław Miłosz, from 'At a Certain Age'

Acknowledgements

Thank you to my agent, Sam Copeland, for believing in my idea. I'm lucky to have had two sensitive, wise and astute editors work with me on the text in Kris Doyle and Ansa Khan Khattak. Thank you to Grace Harrison for how passionately she launched my book into the world and to Emma Bravo and Kieran Sangha for continuing in that spirit, helping to open new doors for me, for which I am very grateful. Thank you to Andrea Henry for her wisdom and her counsel when envisioning the paperback. The whole Picador team have been so welcoming of me and excited about the book and that helped to give me the extra courage I needed to write this story.

I'm grateful to those who have helped me teaching in prisons: Mike Coxhead, Andrea Fassolas, Peter Worley, Emma Worley, Kirstine Szifris, George Pugh, Jose Aguiar and Helena Baptista. Thank you to those who have helped to fund some of my work, such as King's College, Philosophy in Prisons and the Royal Institute of Philosophy.

Thank you to Robert Ellis and Viryanaya Ellis for teaching me so much and for their friendship.

So many writers, artists, journalists and academics gave me their time to help me with my research: Darren Chetty, Iwona Luszowicz, Peter Worley, Lucy Baldwin, Pieter Mostert,

Liviu Alexandrescu, Rachel Tynan, Alice Levins, Laura D'Olimpio, Steve Lowe, Bettina Joy De Guzman, David Breakspear, Yvonne Jewkes, Joanna Pocock, Christopher Impey, Kate Herrity, Jason Warr, Joanna Lear, Sarah Fine, Jamie Lombardi, David Kendall and Jason Buckley.

Thank you to the friends that have been there for me either when I was a kid, at university, when I first started writing or when I was working on this book: Alexandra, Taf, Simon B, Steven CH, Lily, Rebecca, Paul, Jessica, Morgan, Kate H, Marsali, Pips, Mike, Liz, David, Vanessa, Will B, Adam, Steve H, Kate B, Pawel, Iona, Christopher, Guillermo, Rob, Rehana, Bruce, Carol, Irian, Simon K, Steven G, Jane, Fiona, Helen, Rosie, Mark, Giacomo, Sophie, Tari, Andy, Alice, Deb, Kevin, Fin, Sofie, Dana, Kate, Eli, Micheal, Manny, Will S, Val, Roger, Hollie and Tommy.

A special thanks to my mum, brother, uncle and sister-in-law for trusting me with their stories.